PRAISE FOR

LOOKING FOR LIONEL

Sharon has produced a beautiful and moving memoir in her new book *Looking for Lionel*.

From a personal viewpoint, I found Sharon's account of her family's difficult journey into the perplexing and challenging world of Alzheimer's disease . . . to be full of vision, clarity and compassion. We can see fragments of light in the darkness, laughter and humour in unexpected situations and the discovery of a new way of loving and understanding . . . Sharon shows us that love ultimately is able to conquer all and with patience, respect and understanding, our loved ones are never totally lost to us. In fact, that it is possible to find what we have always been looking for.

Marie Phillips

Page by page, with tears and laughter, I read Sharon Snir's moving memoir *Looking for Lionel*, and all the time, I felt myself looking for validation that I had done the right thing with my own dad, as he too faded away to the place Alzheimer's takes our loved ones. With incredible insight, with loving humour and the devotion of an incredible daughter, Sharon has showed us how life can make sense in a senseless disease.

I wish I had this book ten years ago, as I muddled my way through the fog, hoping I was doing the right thing, even when family members disagreed . . . *Looking for Lionel* is a roadmap to anyone travelling this same path. Those that have been touched with Alzheimer's know the pain of the journey, the embarrassment of trying to take them out in public, and the friends that fall along the way. A must for families and anyone that takes care of our mothers, fathers, brothers and sisters.

Judy Robertson, artist and writer

SHARON SNIR

Looking FOR LIONEL

How I lost and found my mother through dementia

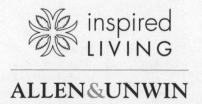

inspired LIVING

ALLEN&UNWIN

Inspired Living, an imprint of
Allen & Unwin
83 Alexander Street
Crows Nest NSW 2065
Australia

Phone: (61 2) 8425 0100
Fax: (61 2) 9906 2218
Email: info@allenandunwin.com
Web: www.allenandunwin.com

Cataloguing-in-Publication details are available
from the National Library of Australia
www.librariesaustralia.nla.gov.au

ISBN 978 1 74175 951 8

Internal design by Christabella Designs
Set in 12/16 pt Bembo by Bookhouse, Sydney
Printed and bound in Australia by Griffin Press

10 9 8 7 6 5 4 3 2 1

Mixed Sources
Product group from well-managed forests, and other controlled sources
www.fsc.org Cert no. SGS-COC-005088
© 1996 Forest Stewardship Council

FSC

The paper in this book is FSC certified. FSC promotes environmentally responsible, socially beneficial and economically viable management of the world's forests.

'. . . people do not consist of memory alone. People have feelings, imagination, drive, will and moral being.'
Cohen and Eisdorfer, *The Loss of Self*, 2001

To my father, Lionel

CONTENTS

FOREWORD BY DR HENRY BRODATY

What struck me about Sharon Snir's roller-coaster account of the twelve-year voyage of Lily, her mother, through dementia is the sensitivity with which she portrays the protagonists in this real-world drama.

As Lily sinks into a world of confusion and dependence, she clutches at her valuables and constantly clings to her security, her husband, Lionel. If he is not there, she searches for him. Lily is looking for Lionel but in the end it is Sharon who finds the person behind the father, the husband and the doctor, and finally establishes a loving relationship with her mother.

Alzheimer's, the most common form of dementia, is a cruel disease. It robs people of their memory, their language, their reasoning and their independence. As the disease progresses it is too easy for others to forget the person camouflaged by the obvious signs of mental decline, and to talk around or to talk down to the affected person. Readers living with loved ones with dementia will recognise how easy it is to fall into these patterns themselves or they may have seen it in how professionals communicate.

On the other hand as we accompany Lily, Lionel and Sharon on their ride, we learn how empathy and understanding can calm agitation and aggression, we learn the importance of considerate communication, we get an idea of how to talk Alzheimer's and we learn the importance of adjusting our rhythm to that of the person with dementia. We also learn that Alzheimer's can strip away the layers of a lifetime of acquired pretensions and habits, and reveal the core of the individual.

Looking for Lionel is about how dementia touches a family's life—there is an aphorism which says 'She has Alzheimer's but they [the family] suffer from it.' I often use the phrase 'dementia touches others', but it is too soft. Dementia thumps, smacks, whacks and hits families' lives for six. We see it here: the dilemma of confronting the diagnosis, the demands and restrictions on families, the emotional turmoils, the ructions between family members over what is best for mum and the anguish of the decision to put mother in a home.

Many, but sadly not all, health professionals are thoughtful and caring. When Lily breaks her hip and goes to hospital, Sharon Snir eloquently captures the nurses' and doctors' lack of understanding of how bewildering the world can be through the fog of dementia.

Looking for Lionel is a good read. The well-known 'downs' of Alzheimer's disease are leavened by many 'ups', and by humour. Along with the dilemmas, and the heartache, we discover much about how best to improve the quality of life for the person with dementia.

Henry Brodaty
Professor of Ageing and Mental Health and
Director, Dementia Collaborative Research Centre,
University of New South Wales, Sydney

FOREWORD BY DEBORAH GLOVER-UETZ

Sharon Snir has shined a light on the often dimly lit topic of Alzheimer's disease and how it affects the individual and their loved ones. Far too often this disease of epidemic proportions is dismissed as a natural part of aging or simple forgetfulness. Even more offensive, it is often the topic of jokes. Those who fail to understand the true nature of an Alzheimer's diagnosis pass it off as an 'old-timers' disease' or 'senior moments'. Those who know the truth about Alzheimer's understand that it is not natural or humorous.

Looking for Lionel lets the story of her mother's illness and the path it followed unfold like a delicate rose. As we become more and more drawn into who this woman was before her illness and who she becomes as it takes a hold upon her, we not only share in the amazing transformations, we also come to understand that everyone who cares about her is also transformed.

Beyond one family's journey through Alzheimer's disease and care giving, we also learn the latest facts and most up-to-date statistics regarding this illness, which now affects millions.

Those who will benefit from this story include medical professionals, who need to understand the human spectrum of their patient's life both before and after diagnosis, as well as those who have already stepped into the world of caregiver, who will be better equipped both emotionally and cerebrally to provide the best world they can for their loved one and accept the new normal.

As the daughter of an Alzheimer's patient I found myself moved to tears, as Lily's journey mirrored my father's. I related deeply to Sharon Snir's description of 'getting the mother she had always wanted' in the ever-changing world of Alzheimer's disease.

The heart, honesty, humour and factual resources found in *Looking for Lionel* make it one of the most important books ever written on the topic. As you travel through the pages let your mind open to all of the wisdom she has imparted. We cannot change what will be with Alzheimer's disease, but changing the way we think of it and react to its challenges can mean the difference between a chaotic existence and a journey that will leave you with precious memories and a deeper understanding of who they were, who they are and who they shall be.

Deborah Glover-Uetz
Author of *Into the Mist: When someone you love has Alzheimer's disease*

INTRODUCTION

Looking for Lionel is a personal story. It is a story of how dementia crept into my family unannounced and left us struggling to hold on to a life that appeared to be slipping away from us like a balloon slipping out of a child's hand. It is a story of fear and courage, shame and pride, sorrow and joy. It is a story of paradox, where the least capable person in our family was, for a time, calling all the shots. It is a story of how our lives changed in ways we never could have imagined.

We learnt a whole new language because the old ways of relating, which required memory, no longer worked. And although dementia is not curable, we discovered it is also not a fate worse than death. This is a story in which, out of the disorder and confusion, the pain and loss, we found the mother we never had.

Dementia is not a disease itself but rather a group of symptoms that may accompany certain brain diseases or conditions. Alzheimer's disease is the most common form of dementia, followed by vascular dementia and frontotemporal dementia or FTD. As our mother, Lily, has both Alzheimer's and vascular dementia, I have chosen to refer to her condition simply as dementia.

Throughout *Looking for Lionel*, I refer to my mother as Lily. It is the name she was given at birth and the name her parents, siblings and school friends always used, but I never heard anyone call her that. She has been known as Leslie for as long as I can remember. I did not even know Lily was her real name until my aunt mentioned it to me about twenty years ago. A strange thing happened, however, when my daughter, now twenty-five, was four years old. Out of the blue one day, she insisted that we call her Lily. She refused to answer to any other name, for one year. Then just as suddenly one day she declared, 'I am not Lily anymore,' and she became Orly again.

1

MY MOTHER, LILY

About twelve years ago my mother began to show signs of dementia. The first signs were so subtle that they were easy to dismiss. Our family did not speak about what was happening for a long time.

Growing up with my mother Lily was not easy. For as long as I can remember she was kind and cruel, sweet and bitter—and stunningly beautiful. The main focus of her world was my father, Lionel, followed by the other essentials of her life: the hairdresser, art, travel, friends, clothes and social events.

Try as I would to be appreciated, accepted and loved by Lily, she rarely showed any interest in me or my sister, Donna, unless we were on 'show'. She had a short temper and would reprimand me regardless of where we were at the time. This only made me try harder to be the child my mother wished for. On the other hand, her friends thought of her as a confidante. To them she was a wise and open-hearted listener, someone who could be trusted with their deepest secrets.

When Lily began to change, naturally her friends did not understand what was happening. Little by little she forgot their names, and the dates and places they planned to meet. She forgot how to turn things on and off. She forgot how to get herself to where she wanted to go and how to get herself back again. She no longer recognised friends and family members. She lost the ability to discuss current events and recent family happenings. She forgot how to play cards, make a pot of tea, and distinguish between an apple and a knife.

Her changes frightened most of her friends away. She began to cry for no particular reason and hung up the phone before conversations were over. Many of her friends were confronted by her behaviour and terrified that if this could happen to Lily, it could happen to them, too. Most of them stopped calling.

These friends who left never got to meet the emerging Lily. Still charming, witty and funny, she had also become softer, and more vulnerable. Never sure what she believed in before, she now knew, without a doubt, that she believed in God and she thanked Him repeatedly every day for the smallest things. Lily now adored every baby that she passed in the street. She lit up every time someone smiled at her and with a childlike innocence warmly acknowledged them as if they were old friends. Those friends who left Lily's life never saw her look deeply into their eyes and tell them, from the heart of her being, that they were so beautiful and that she loved them.

The changes became more noticeable. Lily began to ring me a few times a day and every conversation began by her asking me what my plans were for the day. At first I would tell her she had just called me and she would contradict me, saying it was the first time she had spoken to me that day. She became frustrated with my father when he would innocently correct her. At first she occasionally forgot someone's name but as dementia progressed she forgot everyone's name, except Lionel's.

After eleven years of caring and covering for Lily, my father, Lionel, suffered a heart attack one day in the synagogue. It was not his time to die, but that was the last day my father ever looked after my mother by himself.

In 2008, there were 227,300 people with dementia in Australia, with the number expected to be 731,000 by 2050 unless there is a medical breakthrough.[1]

2

REACTIONS TO ALZHEIMER'S

Some people tend to respond to Alzheimer's and other forms of dementia by pretending it is not really happening. They dismiss the signs with such comments as, 'Oh, she's been forgetful all her life' or 'He has always been a scatterbrain. It's nothing to worry about.'

'I forget things too. You are fine. It's okay.'

Or people believe this is a condition that needs to be understood. They feel more must be done and find ways they can help. They look for solutions to the problems that arise. They organise petitions to build more special care residential homes. They write books about dementia, choose to become geriatrics professionals to help these people live with dignity. They become advocates and activists who fight for the rights of the elderly and those with dementia.

Then there are those who see Alzheimer's as something shameful, and even disgusting. They feel that if someone shows the signs of dementia they should be put away somewhere safe where they cannot disturb or upset anyone.

It is estimated that 35.6 million people worldwide will be living with dementia in 2010. This number will almost double every 20 years, to 65.7 million in 2030 and 115.4 million in 2050.[2]

Understandably, a lot of us are afraid of Alzheimer's. It is unknown territory, a journey without a chance of any U-turns. It's natural to ask, 'What if it happened to me? What if it happens to someone I love. How would I cope?'

Mum's friend, Tracy, would ask me how my mother was whenever she saw me. I would tell her that Mum was fine, healthy—but that she had been forgetting where she parked her car or left her handbag, and that she would get very upset when such incidents happened. 'Your father should put her into a home and get on with his own life,' she would say brusquely. She rarely called Mum anymore. Like many others, she no doubt found Mum's dementia off-putting and confronting.

Until dementia touched my life, I knew very little about the condition. It has been for me a transition from ignorance to knowledge, from grief to acceptance, from sorrow to joy and from fear to love.

3.

SCARED ABOUT DEMENTIA

Just the mention of dementia or Alzheimer's has the power to make the calmest of people shudder. Simple lapses like forgetting to pick up the milk on the way home, not remembering the name of an old friend, or walking into a room and realising we have no idea why we are there, can push a panic button, leaving us with thoughts of dread: 'Oh my God, I think I'm getting Alzheimer's' or 'I hope I'm not getting you-know-what.'

Telltale signs

Whilst writing this book I interviewed almost 30 individuals who knew someone with dementia. Roberta was one of them. She told me she felt she was already following in her mother's footsteps. 'I do suspect I will get it because I already see the same signs in myself . . . I am 52 next month and I can see . . . the same signs I saw in my mother when she was this age. I used to have a photographic memory . . . I don't have that memory anymore and I even feel confused about things that I was very confident about previously. I do suspect that I may be on the same path. I haven't done anything about it. But I have heard there is now a blood test that will be able to tell if I have the propensity for dementia and I am definitely going to do that test.'

Embracing the present

Anne also has some fear she may get Alzheimer's, having also watched her mother go down this road. However, her philosophy is '. . . to be the best, friend, wife, mother, human being I can and to like who I am. I think that is so important. I'm determined to enjoy myself while I can. I keep myself busy. I love music, for example, and sing twice a week . . . I think as long as I seize the day and make sure I have a fulfilling life I am going to use every moment I can in living my life, to the fullest.'

A senior moment?

Every time Lily forgot something she would jokingly say, 'I must be getting Alzheimer's.' How or why she got Alzheimer's I cannot say. However, she certainly thought about it a long time before it became a reality.

Some people couch their fear in more politically appropriate language such as, 'I am having a senior moment' or 'Don't mind me, it's just menopause.' Nevertheless, when we pass a certain age and forget something, many of us fear it is the big 'A'.

Forgetfulness pure and simple

When we get confused we can step into fearful fantasies that we might be getting Alzheimer's and worry about what that will mean for us, our work, our family and friends. It is important, though, to remember that most of us will not get Alzheimer's disease.

Although Alzheimer's disease often begins with a loss of memory, forgetting things does not mean we have Alzheimer's.

I am of the belief that the more we focus on something negative, the more likely we are to create it. Lily had been forgetting things for as long as I can remember her, yet she did not have Alzheimer's when she was thirty or forty years old. So what was it that caused her to be forgetful earlier in her adult life? I can only surmise that with her very busy life, work and social commitments taking up every minute of her day, she never allowed herself to stop, take a few long breaths, become still. I imagine she was rarely really present. Neither my sister nor I can remember a time where Lily sat down and listened to music, for example. She never took a minute to contemplate, to meditate. Everyone who lives this way, whose thoughts are scattered and unfocused, will inevitably forget things. That does not mean they will get Alzheimer's.

Not everyone who jokes, 'I must be getting Alzheimer's' does so.

But if we focus on disease we may help create disease. If we focus on arguing, we tend to create more arguing. Of course, this works in both directions: if we focus on peace, we create peace. If we focus on compassion and love, we help create more compassion and love. Whether Lily was destined to get Alzheimer's, I don't know. However, I am certain that her worry about this possibility over the years didn't help.

4
•

PROTEIN, PLAQUES AND TANGLES

So, how do you know you, or someone you love, has Alzheimer's? First your doctor will rule out other brain or medical problems before they focus on a diagnosis of Alzheimer's disease. By using brain and psychological testing, brain imaging, and other techniques they can determine if someone has:

- probable Alzheimer's disease—the person has no other illnesses that may contribute to the symptoms
- possible Alzheimer's disease—the person meets the criteria for other illnesses that may contribute to his or her mental problems.

I found it interesting to learn that a definitive diagnosis of Alzheimer's can only be made after the person is dead. An autopsy of a brain affected by Alzheimer's reveals distinctive changes. There is an accumulation of a protein substance in the form of plaques, or clumps of fibres, in the brain's grey matter. These plaques contain a hard, waxy deposit that affects the blood vessels around the brain.

Another characteristic of a brain affected by Alzheimer's is tangles within someone's neurons composed of an abnormal form of protein. We need our neurons—cells in our nerve tissue—to process and transmit information. Sensory neurons, for example, respond to touch, sound, and light and then send signals to the spinal cord and brain. Motor neurons receive signals from the brain and spinal cord and send messages to our muscles when we need to move. Scientists believe that the plaques and tangles cause neurons to shrink and eventually die, first in the memory and language centres of the brain, and finally throughout the brain. Sometimes the process can take seven to ten years or even longer. And sometimes there is a rapid deterioration.

This happened to the father of Greg, one of the people I interviewed. 'Dad was not only a busy family doctor but taught medicine at the university for thirty years. He loved his work so much we used to joke that he was married to medicine and we were just a pleasant distraction. When he started to forget patients' histories and struggle with answering students' questions we knew something was wrong. In retrospect it all happened very quickly. He stopped work and almost at the same time stopped talking. In less than three years he couldn't walk without help and lost the ability to feed himself. He always smiled, though. Even when his face could no longer show any emotion, if I waited long enough, I could see it in his eyes.'

5.

DEMENTIA IS A TRANSITION

So what is dementia in practical terms? Basically, dementia is a transition. When a wife can no longer look after herself or a father no longer remembers how he once interacted with other family members. When a friend can no longer remember our name. When a work mate no longer knows who we are. And in response we, too, begin to change.

Initially we try to hold on to what we know. We correct our husband when he makes a mistake. We disagree with our friend when they are telling a story. We confront our loved one when they lose our keys. We get angry when our mother forgets to meet us or our wife hides our laptop computer. Some of us try to cover up. Some of us pretend this is not really happening. Some of us talk about it to everyone we know and some of us tell no one.

Reality check

Whatever the case, dementia always holds up a mirror and reflects back all our fears and insecurities. It is then that we can begin to examine our own behaviour, our own attitudes, and our own judgments. We can, if we choose, be brave and face what is happening right now and let go of what we want to happen. We can become aware of who we are at present—feeling fragile, wondering how we'll cope, angry this is happening to someone we love, terrified about the changes this will bring.

Letting go

Coping with someone with Alzheimer's is exacting. It helps to begin the journey by letting go of past baggage, old resentments and hurts. One of the first places many people turn to get help is their local Alzheimer's Association.[3] These centres, located in most cities around the world, are staffed by social workers, counsellors and experts in the field. They not only understand the problems associated with Alzheimer's but offer support groups, and individual counselling if necessary.

Some people also feel comfortable talking things over with a minister or priest and others choose to confide in close friends. Although reaching out at a time like this can be difficult, realising we are not alone can make the world of difference.

Letting go of past hurts frees us to be in the present moment.

If we choose, we can allow dementia to reconnect us to the only thing that is real, and that is this present moment. Serina, whose father died recently, describes this so well. 'Dad was a grumpy man most of his life. It was never easy for me to be with him. Alzheimer's just exaggerated it even more. There was a lot of yelling during those last years. My mum trying to correct my dad, my sister defending her son whom Dad seemed to always pick on. But I finally got to spend some time with my dad. He would sit with me and talk. I would take him on a daily ride around town . . . always the same route . . . always the same conversation, never changing. Mum would ask me how I could sit with him for so long and I told her I just had patience. I wasn't looking after him all the time like her. But what I really wanted to say was . . .

finally, this man I call Dad is noticing me. But now that he has been gone a few years, I think I was noticing him more.'

When Serina was with her father she was not thinking of other things. When we allow ourselves to fully see and hear and be with our loved one, the relationship becomes a heart-to-heart experience. Serina was not concerned with doing or saying the 'right' thing. Her purpose was to be with her father in whatever way he wanted. Even when our loved one is agitated, delusional or upset, when we let go of how they should be, we can embrace them exactly as they are.

For those who have dementia it can be a transition from being the one everyone depends on, to becoming dependent on everyone.

More than one million Australians are involved in caring for someone with dementia.[4] Understandably, this results in significant strain on families and carers as they struggle to deal with the daily challenges that arise when a loved one has dementia.

Claire's dad did not believe in asking anyone for help. She told me, 'He had come to stay for a few days and was getting ready to go to bed. He had been in the bathroom and was trying to get into his pyjamas. I heard him call me so I went in. There he was, all tangled up in his pyjamas and in his gruff voice he said that he didn't know how to get into these stupid things. I told him the way they make pyjama pants nowadays is ridiculous. I told him not to worry and I bent down and helped him to put them on. He started to cry and whispered he never thought this would happen to him.

'I started to cry with him, then he looked into my eyes and asked me whether he had been a good father. I told him he had been the best. He nodded again and I felt he believed me.'

For some, it is a transition from the fear of life, death, failure or success, to simple acceptance that this is to be their new journey. For some people it is a transition from being attached to the material world to reconnecting to their soul.

6

DEMENTIA AND THE SOUL

In his book *Care of the Soul*, Thomas Moore says the soul is not a thing but a quality or dimension of experiencing life and ourselves. He says the soul is about depth, value, relatedness, heart, personal substance. As I watch my sister, Donna, stroke Lily's cheeks and sing the songs that Lily has always loved, I know they're talking, soul to soul. When Lionel rubs cream on Lily's arms, I no longer see my parents, but two humans who are truly together. When I see a grandchild sitting on the lap of her grandmother who has Alzheimer's, I know that moment may become a memory that touches the child's soul for the rest of their life.

In *Archetypal Psychology,* James Hillman reminds us that our psychology and soul are intrinsically connected by the fact that the word 'psychology' means the 'reason or speech or intelligible account of the soul'. He adds that the soul has a way of bringing out everything that is profound, mysterious and confusing about life.[5]

By being fully with our loved one on their journey moment by moment, we become two souls connecting rather than missing each other.

Psychotherapist Dr Dan Gottlieb sums this up well:

You (caregiver) do not suffer because of them [person with dementia]. They have a disease, a neurological illness, that's a fact. But that's not why you suffer. You suffer because you love. If you did not love, you would not suffer. And the more you love, the more you suffer. Problem is, when you try to do something you cannot do, or be something you cannot be, the guilt, shame, anxiety and fear makes the love go underground . . . and you can't feel the love anymore. Love is learning to live with your helplessness in the face of your loved one's suffering.[6]

Put simply, dementia is the opportunity to move from conditional to unconditional love. This is something dementia has taught me. Lily was very much a physical person. She sped around the local sports oval at six o'clock every morning, with Lionel. Lionel would proudly joke that it was getting harder and harder to keep up with her. Appearance to Lily was all-important. She was concerned about the appearance of her home. The cushions in our lounge room had to be fluffed up just so. God help anyone who sat on them. They were to look at, not to sit on! If we ever dropped a crumb onto the floor, she would run to the broom cupboard, take out the dustpan and sweeper and clean it up, along with a large portion of the surrounding floor. She expected her two daughters to look a certain way, especially slim. Unlike most 'Jewish mothers' instead of offering me a little more to eat she would whisper in my ear, 'Darling, do you really need to eat that?'

'The human heart yearns for contact . . . each of us secretly and desperately yearns to be met,' says therapist Richard Hycner.[7] Every child needs to be able to walk into a room and have a parent light up, just because they are, and for no other reason. Indeed, we all need to feel that we are of value simply because we are. During my childhood I walked on shaky ground around my mother. I wanted her to see me, to acknowledge me, to admire me and to approve of me. The more I tried to be the person I thought she wanted, the less interested in me she became.

After I left home, married, travelled and lived abroad I had five children and was well on the way to letting go of the possibility of having the mother I had always wanted. By the time I had completed my studies in psychotherapy, I had learnt that while I might not have had the mother I wanted, I had the mother I needed.

I realised her inability to love me the way I wanted was not about me at all. As I learnt to accept and love myself unconditionally, I began to accept and love Lily unconditionally also.

Dementia peeled away layers of how things should and should not be. It peeled away the surface that was concerned only with appearance. Over time it revealed someone I had never really met. Someone pure and sweet and filled with innocent gratitude. In the end, all that was left of Lily was Love. How ironic that dementia gave me the mother I had always wanted.

As dementia progressed, she declared her love and joy at being with me every time we met. She looked into my eyes and often cried. I would ask her, 'Why are you crying, Mama?' And she would try to explain, but all she could say was, 'I love you. You are my life.' And she would hold me and cry on my shoulder.

L+L

Lily always knew my face but she no longer knew that I was her daughter.

I once asked Lily how old she was and she told me, 'Twenty-three.' That being her perception, of course she could not possibly know me as her daughter. All the same, I often told her that she was my mother. 'Do you know why I call you Mummy?' I asked her.

She looked at me in silence. I continued, 'Because you are my mummy and I am your daughter. I am Sharon.' Then she threw her thin little arms around me and said, 'Oh! I didn't know. Thank you, thank you for telling me. I will never forget that.'

It is no longer important whether Lily knows who I am, only that I love her.

The day someone is diagnosed with any form of dementia is the day everyone in that family knows life will never be the same again. Once dementia is diagnosed there is no turning back. The disease will eventually take away most of the cognitive and eventually the physical abilities of your loved one. And yet loss is far from the whole story. The journey is like a labyrinth and every corner reveals a hidden gift. You only have to look.

7
.

LOSING DAVID

On a freezing cold Sunday, in Glasgow, on 4 December 1927, Lily Joseph arrived in the world. A brother and two sisters waited at home to hear the news of her birth. She grew up in Scotland, as did her father before her.

Her mother, Leah, was born in Riga, in Latvia. In the spring of 1915, the German army defeated the Russian army and forced it to retreat from Poland and Lithuania. People began to spread rumours that Jews were spying for Germany and were responsible for the German victory. Under duress or voluntarily, about 127,000 Jews left Latvia during the war.

Leah, Lily's mother, was put on a ship by her parents. They knew this was the only way to protect their children from the violent pogroms—organised massacres—of Jews in Latvia at that time. With their last roubles, Leah's parents bought passage for their eight children to America. They were not able to travel together, but they prayed they would meet again soon. Leah was the last to leave. Her distraught mother gave her one final word of advice. 'When you board the ship, my darling, do not look back. Just look forward. Look towards America.' But of course she turned around just as her mother collapsed in unbearable grief on the dock. That image remained with her all her life. She never saw her parents again and the ship did not go to America.

For some reason the captain changed the destination of the ship and a few weeks later, they docked in Glasgow, Scotland. I can't imagine how Leah must have felt, all alone in a strange land. But she was a strong woman and within two years she met a man who was to become her husband. His name was David.

Lily adored her father, David. He favoured and spoiled his baby daughter long after she had grown up.

A year after the Second World War ended, David developed a tumour on the brain. Perhaps it was the result of an injury he sustained in combat during the war; we will never know. But when he was taken to hospital no one imagined the end was so near.

Lily was now twenty-two years old and for her the world was bubbling with postwar frivolity. She wanted to celebrate. She wanted go out and party and 'kick up her heels'. And when David became ill, Lily thought it was a passing malady.

David began to deteriorate quickly. Lily refused to listen to her sisters when they told her that David wanted to see her. Lily accused them of making a mountain out of a molehill. She told them she would visit him. Soon.

Lily held fast to her denial that her father was dying. She distracted herself with everything she had missed during the war. Perhaps for Lily 'out of sight' was really 'out of mind'. I will never know. I can only imagine, knowing my mother, that she probably thought if she ignored the whole situation, it would go away. Of course the situation didn't go away. David died and Lily never said goodbye.

Guilt is an insidious emotion. Like a fungus, it grows in the dark and spreads throughout one's whole existence. Day after day, Lily thought she heard her father calling her. She would run into his room looking for him. She would wake up at night hearing his voice and jump out of bed, only to find the house dark and quiet. She thought she was going insane.

It was decided she needed a holiday. She would travel on the *Orion* to Australia and visit her aunt who lived in Sydney. No one really knows what happened on that ship, but when Lily disembarked, she had changed her name and her age. She stepped onto Australian soil with a completely new identity. No one ever called her Lily again, not until one September afternoon, on the day she moved into a Residential Care Unit for people with dementia.

8
.

I'M LILY

Soon after my mother became a resident at the Residential Care Unit, she and my father, Lionel, were walking in the garden, and they sat down on a wooden seat next to some beautiful white flowers. Lionel pointed to the flowers and commented that they were lilies. Although he knew Lily had changed her name so many years ago, they had never discussed it. It was completely taboo. Lily laughed and said casually, 'Like me. I'm Lily.' If it wasn't traumatic enough to bring his beautiful wife to live in the Residential Care Unit it almost knocked him to the ground to hear her say that!

Throughout my life, my mother has been distracted. Although there was always a gaiety and glamour about her, I cannot remember ever having a deep conversation with her. She literally never sat still long enough. I worried that leaving her adoring husband of fifty-five years, her home and everything that was familiar to her would kill her. Instead, it cracked open some invisible concrete casing that protectively held the real and exquisitely beautiful woman once called Lily.

Lily has softened into the mother I always wanted. She looks into my eyes as I cup her cheeks and tell her that I love her.

Every time I visit her she tells me how beautiful I am and how I am her life. She helps Dorothy, the woman who works in the kitchen, serve breakfast and lunch every day. She tells the maintenance man that she loves him, and she does. She cries with delight every time I arrive, and although she does not know my name, she knows she loves me, and for me that is enough.

Dementia not only changes our loved one but it irrevocably alters our relationship with them. Anne, whose mother, Monique, has dementia, had long accepted that her relationship with her mother was never going to be as close as she would have liked. When Monique developed dementia, she told me, 'I didn't expect for my mum to lose her aggressive edge and for me to like her a whole lot more than when I was growing up and I think that is a great blessing. And now, because she lives in a facility that does respect my mother's dignity I really appreciate every moment I spend with her. I really feel blessed to have been given this opportunity to enjoy my mother in a way I never did before.'

Dementia is a major determining factor in precipitating entry to residential care. At least 60 per cent of people in high-care facilities and 30 per cent of people in low-care facilities have dementia. Many more have an obvious cognitive impairment (90 per cent high care; 54 per cent low care).[8]

9
.

IF YOU KNEW CHAOS
LIKE I KNEW CHAOS

Lily flourished on inconsistency. She adored her friends, yet often ignored her children. She was a marvellous cook, yet we rarely shared a meal together. She was overprotective to the point that she would walk into the school locker room mid-morning to tie my sports shoelaces yet she would leave us for months on end while she was travelling overseas. She was warm, loving and proud of us when we were dressed up like dolls and paraded in front of her friends yet if we spoke up or gave our opinion she would become wild with anger. I think I must have been the only child forbidden to make my own bed. For as long as I can remember, that was the job of the live-in housekeeper.

A succession of housekeepers slept in the small yellow room off the kitchen and I hated them all. They each brought with them their own unique and, to me, sickly smell, which would waft into the kitchen from that bedroom. They were supposed to be mother's helpers but I wanted my mother, not her helper.

Their chores included bringing tea and toast to my mother's bed every morning, making all the beds, washing and ironing, cleaning the house and preparing our breakfast and packing school lunches.

Every few months a new woman would arrive at our home. There was an interview process, which I was never allowed to attend, but would listen to as I pressed my ear to the door, holding my breath till I felt myself go weak at the knees with lack of oxygen. Some of the women left after only a few weeks. In those days pregnant country girls would come to work in the city as domestics and mother's helpers until their babies were due to be born.

Magda, however, was not pregnant, and her existence was the bane of my eight-year-old life. She did everything she was told to do. She made my mother her breakfast tray every morning. She tidied up after us and put our toys and clothes away. My mother had no complaints. But I did.

Magda would criticise my mother ruthlessly behind her back and my cheeks would burn with shame. She would tell me how incompetent, spoilt and indulged my mother was. When Lily went out she would say things under her breath as she made my afternoon tea. I caught muttered phrases like, *She should be doing this*, *hopeless woman*, and I would overhear her talking on the phone splashing her sentences with words such as *witch*, *evil*, *ugly* and *ungrateful*.

Each day, perfect squares of Vegemite and peanut butter sandwiches appeared on the table in front of me.

It was all so neat.

That was the way my mother liked it. Her bedroom was her boudoir and I was not allowed inside unless she was with me. She had a beautiful vanity table with a huge ornate mirror. She would sit on the small tapestry-covered stool perched in front of the mirror when she put on her makeup. Gorgeous dresses, hand-beaded with pearls and sequins hung on rainbow hangers. Elegant coats and furs draped the coat hangers, and shoes to match her day and evening garments lined the floor of her polished wooden wardrobe.

Every day at five o'clock my mother briskly walked down the hall to prepare for my father's arrival home. It was a ritual, a sacred ritual that included four to five sweeping brushstrokes to freshen her hair, a spray of perfume into the air above her head and the luscious layering of red, pink or apricot lipstick on the bottom lip only. Then she would smooch her lips together and look briefly in the mirror and at the same time the sound of my father's keys opening the front door would be heard.

A bottle of red wine stands half empty outside on the weathered table, and Lionel is heaving a familiar sigh of tired frustration. We are planning to go out for a bite to eat and Lily has lost her handbag. Gradually he stands up, round-shouldered, head bent strangely forward, perhaps an indication of stress, and slowly begins the search. Usually her bag is in the most unlikely place. He moves the bed, looks behind cushions, peeks in the laundry, opens the washing machine, and all the while he sighs and shakes his head. From where I am sitting I can hear a t–t–t sound as he sucks his tongue behind his teeth. I begin to stand up to look with him and my mum grabs my arm. Lily has worn the same track pants for three days and her t-shirt is stained with something I can't distinguish.

I try again and suddenly my mother yells at me, 'Where are you going?' I tell her I want to help Lionel find her bag. She pushes me back onto the chair saying, 'I'll find it. You stay there.' I want to help her but she is furious now.

I sit back down and wait. I look at the old pendulum clock hanging on the wall. Five o'clock. I begin to walk down the hall into my mum and Lionel's room. Piles of shoes are heaped under the small glass table in front of the couch. The bed is a patchwork of underwear, tissues, and skirts on coat hangers, old jumpers and lipsticks.

Both my parents are agitated and upset. Lily is running around desperately trying to find something, but she has forgotten what.

Lionel is clearly close to his wits' end. He remembers Lily stuffed her bag with money and precious jewellery earlier that day. I want to scream, *Why don't you just flush it all down the toilet! It's the same thing. You let her stuff your hard-earned money into her bag and she goes out and leaves it somewhere.* I want to yell at him, *Why don't you hide all her precious things? Why don't you stop her?*

But I know he can't stop her. He can't. It's too invasive. Too frightening. Too dangerous. There is a great big fat secret in our family. We don't discuss 'it'. We don't address 'it'. We walk around, tiptoe over 'it' and pretend to ignore 'it'.

But it is blatantly obvious that Lily has dementia. She has not been assessed. To arrange an assessment would require something to be said to her and one of the 'rules' is that we are not allowed to say anything that might upset her.

Lionel finds the bag. It is hanging on a coat hanger in a wardrobe. The money is gone. So are the tissue parcels that held gold earrings, a diamond ring and a lovely pearl necklace. Gone. Just gone.

In their place, however, are ten lipsticks. All without their lids. All squashed and slippery inside the bag. Some of them look like they have been 'borrowed' from the display counter of the local department store, others look as if they came from the drawer in my mother's vanity table from long ago.

As those we love slip away from us, tiny shared rituals they loved in the past will bridge the gap.

I gently link my arm with hers and suggest we go put on some lipstick and glam ourselves up a bit. We walk into the bathroom and, with great care, I glide the shapeless lipstick across her bottom lip. She smooches her lips together and there, like magic, my mother is the most beautiful woman in the world again.

Justine's husband is only in his fifties and has been diagnosed with early onset of Alzheimer's. She told me, 'He doesn't realise how bad he is until he does something very obvious and then he gets very upset. He has cycles of going along very well and then something happens and he gets argumentative and eventually has a bit of a cry and everything is fine again. For a while. He is really into denial. He says I am exaggerating. It's very difficult. He knows he has it but he doesn't think anyone notices.'

Broadly speaking there are four stages of dementia: pre, early, moderate and severe. In the first two stages people begin to suspect something is not quite right. They will begin to feel frightened and even embarrassed that their memory is 'playing up'.

They will fight to keep up the façade of being in control, making up a story to fill the gap when they can't remember, or changing the subject when asked a question, or denying they had anything to do with a lost object is considered normal for people in the early stages of dementia. Anything to hold onto a small piece of control. This is a most frightening and difficult stage for both the person with dementia and their loved ones.

The need to still know what is going on leads people with stage one dementia to ask the same questions over and over again. They will use every opportunity to exercise the control they feel they are losing. They will blame others for their memory lapses and unless we understand this we can take their accusations personally. But what they are doing is trying with every fibre of their being not to lose control over their own lives.

By the time they move into the second stage of dementia people are more inclined to relax and give in or let go a little more.

10
·

OH DEAR, WHAT CAN
THE MATTER BE?

Children were arriving, carrying presents for our twin boys. The house was decorated with blue, green and turquoise streamers and yellow balloons. Sandwiches, meat pies, sausage rolls, tomato sauce, fairy bread and plastic baskets of potato chips were arranged on the dining room table. And of course two cakes—one shaped like a soccer field and one looking like a blue swimming pool—were hidden in the pantry awaiting their grand entrance.

Lily and Lionel arrived, carrying presents and a bottle of wine. By eight o'clock that morning, Lily had already phoned me twice, the first time to ask me what I was doing today, the second time to tell me it had been a long time since we had last spoken.

As soon as Lily arrived, she wanted to know what she could do to help. She always wanted to help. The problem was that Lily's 'help' lately was more of a hindrance. She was prone to breaking things, and I noticed that when I asked her to wash up for me, she would hurriedly rinse the dirty plates and put them away in strange places. I had found a plate in the garbage and cutlery in the fridge. I already had my hands full with the twins' seventh birthday party, and twenty-five children piling into the house. I just didn't have the patience to find her something to do. I snapped at her to please sit down and she got angry with me, complaining loudly to Lionel, 'It seems I can't do anything right!'

I immediately felt guilty and told her that as soon as everyone had arrived, she could help carry the plates outside. 'Okay. You just let me know and I'll be there.'

She turned to find Lionel and saw another guest, a young man named Sam. The conversation was clear and simple.

'Hello.' She introduced herself, and asked, 'How are you?'

'Fine, thanks.'

'What's your name?'

'Sam.'

Sam was going out with our eldest daughter, Sheli. He was sixteen and trying to look cool and comfortable. He chatted with Lily for a minute, excused himself and walked over to Sheli, who was busy greeting a group of boisterous seven-year-old boys who had all arrived together.

Lily asked me again what she could do to help and I asked her to take the bowl of potato chips to the table. She spun around towards the veranda where all the children were playing and I was about to tell her that the chips were in the kitchen when she stopped next to Sam. Clearly not remembering she had just spoken to him, she began the same conversation that they had just finished. Sam looked flustered and embarrassed and squeezed out a 'Hi.'

I, too, was embarrassed. I felt ashamed to be embarrassed by my own mother, but I was. I gently took hold of her arm and guided her away. I reminded her that Sam was Sheli's boyfriend and with some desperation added, 'You remember him, don't you?'

She pulled her arm away from me and marched into the kitchen, all the time mumbling, 'Of course I remember him.' Clearly irritated, she started washing some of the clean dishes. One slipped out of her hand and smashed onto the floor. I couldn't stop myself. I yelled at her and told her to leave the dishes and come outside.

I caught a worried glance from my sister, Donna. A silent acknowledgment that something was wrong. Was it possible that Lily was—it felt a betrayal to even think the word—getting dementia? It was becoming more and more clear that she was not herself. Sometimes she forgot where she had been during the day. Occasionally she would lose her car keys, which was less of a problem—they always turned up—but recently she had been forgetting where she'd parked her car. Lionel would then have to drive around the shops until he found it.

I think we knew, but we both sensed it was forbidden to say it out loud. Indeed, nothing would be said for a very long time. Donna took Lily by the arm and led her into the kitchen. They carried the food to the table and in her usual warm and friendly manner, Lily chatted with everyone. Her repertoire was fairly standard.

'Darling, you look wonderful. I love your hair' (substitute with dress, shirt, makeup, tan, shoes . . .).

Madeleine, my cousin, walked over to Lily and commented how fast time flies. 'It is amazing the twins are already seven.'

Lily looked deeply into Madeleine's brown eyes and said, 'You have such lovely skin. Whatever you're doing, don't stop.' Madeleine nodded and hugged Lily. I wondered how long Lily had been saying that line. *Whatever you're doing, don't stop.* It was her signature sentence. Every time she said it, people laughed and every time people laughed Lily knew everything was all right. Lily was a master of making light of any situation. She covered up for her fading memory by being charming and lighthearted.

Things were far worse at home than any of us realised. Lionel felt no one really understood. 'I think the family knew there was a problem but they didn't know how difficult it was. There was a continuous need to watch her. She couldn't even make a cup of tea in the morning. She had lost the ability to cook and I don't think the family really knew what was going on. I think most people found her amusing. If you asked her to get a glass of water she would come back with a bottle of vodka. It wasn't amusing for me. I lived with her and the family didn't.'

Later that afternoon, Sheli and I carried the two candlelit birthday cakes outside. The twins stood side by side and we sang to each of them. Lily walked up and I put my arm around her. Maybe all this was just my imagination. Maybe she was just being her scatty self. Then, Lily glanced at Sam from the corner of her eye and whispered to me, 'That's a nice-looking boy. What's his name?'

I stared at her and slowly whispered, 'That's Sam. He is Sheli's boyfriend.'

Then I saw it in her face. It was so fleeting that I doubt anyone else would have noticed it. It began in her eyes, a blink, and then she swallowed. In one lucid moment, like a sword slicing through soft flesh, she remembered she had already met Sam. She knew, in one appalling instant that something was wrong with her.

She spun around, strode over to Lionel and demanded he take her home. I wanted to tell her that everything would be fine. I wanted to apologise for being irritated, that the dish she had dropped meant nothing at all to me. I wanted to hug her and hold her and make her believe that nothing was wrong.

She repeated, more insistently this time. 'Lionel, I want to go home—now.' Lionel nodded resignedly. I walked them slowly down the driveway and wondered if things would ever be the same again.

11

·

WHERE, WHERE, WHERE CAN IT BE?

Lily would hide her bag in obscure places and when the time came to go out, it could not be found. Life became punctuated by a series of lost objects. Lionel would look all over the house and gradually become more and more stressed and upset. Lily would look, too. She looked in her wardrobe, noticed a shirt, took it out, placed it on the bed, turned around, noticed some shoes, carried them to the bathroom, noticed the toothpaste and brought it into her bedroom and noticed her gloves and perfume, took them out and put them under a pillow and so on.

Then Lionel would ask her if she remembered where she left her bag and of course she would start looking again and notice something else and so on until Oren, my husband, would arrive to pick them up and bring them to our house for dinner. Or until Lionel stopped the whole chaotic charade and suggested they have a glass of wine. That always worked.

Lionel would open their daily bottle of red wine around 5.30 every evening and for about an hour they drank together, and the tears of despair would dry up and they would enjoy each other and remember snippets of the good old times. Lily would repeat a word or a phrase over and over and Lionel would respond with infinite patience, often trying to unravel the thoughts that Lily was no longer able to express. He didn't mind. He enjoyed those times together with his beloved Lily. Sometimes they would go out for dinner and sometimes the bottle of wine would replace dinner and Lily would fall onto her bed, fully dressed until morning. This had never happened before and as we assumed it happened very rarely we did not worry.

Those evening drinks became Lily's favourite time of the day.

It was not until we realised Lily and Lionel were losing weight that we thought to ask whether they were eating. It was then that we learnt about the occasions where they would both fall into bed after a bottle of wine, without having eaten anything except a few chips and savoury dips. I wouldn't have begrudged her that time for the world, but later we all paid the price. Especially Lily.

12

•

FRIGHTENED FRIENDS

Lily and I were walking together in the street where she had lived and worked for many years. She greeted every person who passed us. 'Hullo. How are you?' People stopped and politely tried to remember where they knew this friendly woman from. 'You look so well,' she said. 'Whatever you are doing, just don't stop!'

Eventually, they went on their way, albeit utterly confused. This continued until I saw Elizabeth, a friend of perhaps forty years, walking towards us. I was about to wave when suddenly she looked up, stopped, turned around and crossed the road. That was the first time. It happened many times after that.

Lionel did his best to maintain old friendships. He called Alana and Peter, and suggested they meet for dinner. Lily was confused and disorientated that night. She could not get dressed alone and refused help from Lionel. By the time they arrived at the restaurant she was very upset. She began to welcome everyone who walked in. She told each person how wonderful it was to see them and invited them to come over and say hello to Lionel. Lionel was unwilling to interrupt her. He knew this would make her even more disorientated, so he paid no heed to what was happening. Each time she returned to the table he warmly included her in the conversation but as soon as the door opened she jumped up again. At one point Alana turned to Lily and said, 'Oh Lily, please do stop doing that. You are embarrassing me.'

One never knows exactly when a mild-mannered man may turn into a ferocious lion. When the glass suddenly shatters into a thousand shards. When the earth cracks open and hot molten rock erupts.

That's what happened to Lionel. He looked directly at Alana and roared, 'How dare you speak to Lily that way! If you are embarrassed, then leave. Go! In fact it is you who is embarrassing me.'

Alana, to her credit, realised Lionel was desperate. He adored Lily. Although she was nothing like the Lily he had married, he loved her and had vowed to protect her always. Alana did not leave. She placed a comforting hand on Lionel's shoulder and apologised. Lily, on the other hand, was having none of that and pushed Alana's hand off, leaned over and kissed Lionel.

From that moment, tears of laughter diluted the atmosphere and the rest of the evening flowed with ease.

Everyone is familiar with the experience of shame. A three-year-old grabbing the wrong hand in the supermarket can feel it. It can be triggered by something as trivial as raising our arm to wave at a friend across the street and then discovering that it is not our friend at all. We avert our eyes, wince and hope no one noticed. Shame can occur with any real or imagined rejection or when a yearning that is deeply private is exposed. We feel shame when we say something we judge as silly or thoughtless or when someone we are intimately connected to says or does something inappropriate.

Dementia triggers shame in a
number of ways. For example the shame we
feel when we are confronted by people with
dementia. We recognise ourselves, disgraced, in
the demented person and then we want to draw
back and keep our distance. We see self-control
and discretion stripped away. As long as
we disown this identification we feel
ashamed to be with them and indeed
ashamed of them.

Then there is the shame we feel in anticipation of something the person may do that leads us to discreetly act in a certain way. Sometimes people are able to empathise deeply with the person with dementia and try to 'cover up'.

Lionel was so exquisitely sensitive to what would shame Lily that his covering for her showed the highest form of respect for her dignity. Another example of this sensitivity is when the staff in nursing homes or institutions realise that the appearance of the residents and their surroundings matter. People with dementia show us the strengths and limits of what we value about our lives. Stephen Post, Peter Whitehouse and Robert Binstock, renowned experts in the field of ageing say, 'We should recognise the dignity of the demented as part of our lives and the lives of those we love and as refracted images of ourselves.'[9]

In talking about her mother, Monique, Anne said, 'The most important aspect of dealing with a parent with dementia is that someone has to take control of the situation, but how you do that is with enormous dignity and kindness and remembering always that . . . [they] cared for you for so many years and now you care for them, keeping their dignity intact. And you have to make decisions for the wellbeing of that person, so every decision you make needs to come from care in maintaining their dignity.'

13

BREAKING THE SILENCE

Lily developed a behaviour that is common in dementia: she would wrap her treasures in pieces of facial tissues and hide them in places around the house. Sometimes the tissues found their way into old handbags, sometimes into potplants, sometimes cupboards. Pottering around the house she would later find these tissues and would throw them all away. Most of her jewellery ended up being flushed down the toilet. We watched and said nothing.

Until one night.

Every week our family ate dinner on Friday night together. Lily and Lionel would arrive early and Donna and her children would turn up just before sunset. On this particular day Lily arrived, clearly upset, and went straight over to our dog, PK, and petted him. Lionel, panting and pale, sat down, placed his head in his hands and for one shocking moment I thought he was going to cry. And then he did. It was a silent sob that wrenched itself up from a crater deep within, a dark and frightening place that I had never connected to my father before. We brought him a glass of wine. He refused it. Oren sat beside him and put a gentle arm around his shoulders.

Lily was in the kitchen feigning busyness. She lifted the lid of the warming pumpkin soup and then turned to rinse a few plates that lay in the sink. I asked her gently if she was okay. She shook her head and I pressed a little more. 'Did you have a fight with Dad?'

'I don't know. I just say something to your father and . . .' A stream of disconnected words, saturated with emotion and devoid of logical connection, poured forth. She was confused, and upset and anxious and tired. So, so, tired. She started to cry and then suddenly stopped and said, 'I'm sorry. I have to stop. Your father. I don't want to upset him.'

I took her by the arm and we joined Lionel and Oren. Our children were sitting around the coffee table. Donna and her children had not yet arrived. No one spoke. It was one of those moments when helplessness seemed to spread out across the room like an insidious fog.

We had never addressed this disease by name. We had been silenced by the unspeakable. Lily shook her head and said, 'I don't know what is happening to me.' I looked around and before I knew it the words tumbled out, 'Mummy, do you want to know what is happening to you?'

'Yes.' She looked at me, pleadingly. 'Tell me.'

Nothing could have been clearer and yet everyone had stopped breathing. I saw Donna walk in and, sensing something, she sat down next to Lionel and took his hand.

I stepped onto the diving board and jumped. 'You have a condition . . . a condition that makes you forget things. You will even forget we had this conversation in a few minutes.' I smiled and she smiled back, nodding and listening with excruciating intensity. Willing herself to hear me and to understand.

'You have a special condition. And what it means is that you never ever need to worry about anything again. Nothing, because we are going to look after you. We are going to remember everything for you from now on. You don't have to be responsible for anything either. We are going to do all that for you because we love you so much. Is that okay?'

She began to cry. 'Thank you. Thank you for telling me. Thank you. I'll never forget you for as long as I live.' She kissed me and one by one we all kissed Lily.

And of course she did forget. It took about thirty seconds before nothing remained in Lily's mind about that conversation, but she was calm. The ripples of that conversation touched everyone in the family and the truth was not nearly as traumatic as any of us had imagined. We had not only survived the 'forbidden conversation' but Lily and Lionel were sitting together on the couch holding hands and leaning into each other, relaxed and happy. I believe that from that moment something in Lily acknowledged she could rest now. The strain of keeping the secret was over and although she physically had forgotten the words I had spoken, she felt safe and protected. More importantly we, as a family, were now free to talk with each other about our own feelings.

14

·

PUTTING THE PAST TO REST

Developmental psychologist Bruno Bettelheim says, 'What cannot be talked about can also not be put to rest; and if it is not, the wounds continue to fester from generation to genera- tion.'[10] 'Talking about our feelings is not complaining. It is giving ourselves permission to express openly, without fear or shame.' As a family we had entered a new phase. We began to talk. This new phase of our lives gave us the courage to explore issues that had never been addressed before. Stories of our childhood, many of which our dad knew nothing about. We shared events we all remembered but now added own personal interpretations. Sometimes we laughed and sometimes we cried.

My sister Donna was born two years and three months after me. Where I was dark-haired and serious, she had soft blonde curls and Shirley Temple dimples. We grew up side by side but rarely played with each other. As sisters, however, we shared a deep connection—a sixth sense, you could say—that enabled us to know and often experience what the other was going through.

As our family moved into this new phase, Donna, Dad and I began to speak to each other about our lives, our hurts and sorrows of the past. Dad shared his own stories and we listened with reverence and wonder. He told us how difficult it was to be born the youngest of six children when his parents were ready to retire. They were both in their fifties and had no interest in another child. He had no memory of ever being told he was loved, much less being shown. He did poorly in school and often would come home to find a note asking him to get his own meals when his parents were away. Eventually he came to realise that there was no one to rely on but himself and decided to become a doctor. He worked hard and began to shine academically. No one ever attended his graduation from school or university. No one in his family ever acknowledged his success and achievements in medicine. The war brought with it a job on a ship as a doctor and that in turn took him to London, where he trained as a surgeon. After completing his surgical fellowship in London he returned to Australia.

All this he did alone. As he was never given anything, he confessed how hard it was for him to know how to give and also how to receive.

'In October of 1952 I married the most beautiful girl in the world,' Lionel told us. 'We had met only nine weeks before and we both knew, almost at once, that we had met our soul mate. Since then there has been hardly a day that we have not walked hand in hand somewhere in this wide, wide world.

'We were so different. She was gorgeous, loquacious, full of life, extroverted, and able to converse with everyone, altogether wonderful. I was quiet, introverted, serious, rather short and thirty-four years old. I had no money. She was at least ten years my junior and I could hardly believe my luck.'

Slowly, by talking with great care and listening with deep respect, the wounds that we had all carried began to heal.

But Lily continued to deteriorate.

15

·

DISCOVERING DESPAIR

At first Lionel welcomed friends phoning and offering to take Lily out for coffee. Hours of caring for her denied him even a moment to himself. She would sit on the peacock-blue vinyl-covered chair in his office and watch him read his emails. He would try to interest her in the emails, reading them to her and talking about the topics that appeared on the screen in front of him, but she quickly lost interest. Sometimes he would ask her to go into the kitchen and bring him an apple, and she would go into the bedroom and look everywhere, having forgotten even before she left Lionel's office what it was she had been asked to do. She would become increasingly angry. She imagined he was having affairs with the people who contacted him. She threatened to leave Lionel a dozen times a day. Sometimes she would walk out the front door and promise never to return. Lionel felt power-less, remaining in his office for a few minutes until he realised she was not coming back. Fearing the worst, he would go out and search for her. Eventually he would find her, wandering lost and confused, and overjoyed to see him. Throwing herself into his arms, she would walk home with him.

'The day she placed a piece of bread on the open flame on the stove to make toast and it caught on fire, I knew I needed help. She sometimes forgot how to light the stove and even if she did remember she would walk away leaving the gas on. I knew it was no longer safe to leave her alone and I desperately needed to have a break. For the first time in my life I started to imagine not having to wake up in the morning.'

So when the phone rang and it was two old friends, Mimi and Robin, inviting Lily for coffee, he gratefully accepted. The problem was, Lily no longer wanted to go anywhere without Lionel. She hung onto him like a vine clinging to an old tree trunk.

No one had any idea how much effort went into getting Lily ready to go out. Lionel helped Lily shower and dress. He would lay out her underwear, socks, pants and shirt neatly on the bed. He would try to put on her makeup. Sometimes, however, Lily put on her own makeup using a biro as an eyebrow pencil. Her surprised friends would then be greeted by Lily sporting bright purple eyebrows. Although Lionel tried to coax her into the mood to go out, he rarely succeeded. By the time the doorbell rang she was often furious, but as soon as the door opened, Lily became her old charming self. She flicked her hair back, took whosever arm was offered and walked out the door as if she had been looking forward to their visit all morning.

Mimi and Robin beamed at Lily as she opened the door. 'Are you ready? We are taking you out for coffee.' Lionel put a hand on Lily's shoulder. 'Off you go, darling. I've got some work to do and I'll be here when you get back.' Lily kissed him warmly and walked out the door, closing it behind her.

Silence. He missed her already.

16

DEMENTIA IS A STIGMA

As time passed, fewer friends called. It was one thing to have purple eyebrows around the house but even the most understanding friends did not know how to handle this out in the street. It was even more challenging when Lily greeted every passer-by with a hug and kiss and then walked away, forgetting who she was having coffee with. Lily loved babies and sometimes she would see a mother carrying her new baby in the street and she would walk up and simply take the baby in her arms because she wanted to hug it. Naturally, this behaviour was shocking to her friends and very difficult to understand.

'We cannot expect [people with dementia] to adjust their needs to our ways; rather we must tune our ways to meet their needs.'[11]

Author Jolene Brackey[12] says the developmental level of someone in the middle stages of Alzheimer's is about eight years old. In her work with people with Alzheimer's she has observed that as the disease progresses the developmental age of the individual decreases. Although that observation is a helpful guideline, I would add that there is a vast difference between children and people with dementia. Jane Verity, CEO of Dementia Care Australia, reminds us that, 'People with dementia have lived a long life and carry a backpack full of life experience, history and wisdom. A child does not have this rich knowledge or experience.' She adds, 'The danger of thinking that a person with dementia becomes like a child is that it is likely to affect your whole attitude and way of speaking and you end up talking down to the person as if he or she were a child.'[13]

People with dementia often lose their inhibitions. If they want something they will often just reach out and take it. They don't have any internal conflict about such an action. The problem is, of course, that unless the person is in an environment where it is understood that this is 'normal behaviour', others are going to react with shock, anger and even fear.

Well-known author Terry Pratchett, OBE, was diagnosed with posterior cortical atrophy or PCA, an uncommon variant of dementia, in 2008. He contrasts the diagnosis of Alzheimer's to cancer: 'If you have cancer then you are a brave battler but when you have Alzheimer's you are an old fart . . . It makes you feel quite alone.'[14] People with dementia often report losing friends after a diagnosis. For the partners and carers of people with dementia this can make life unbearably lonely.

Lily started to say whatever she thought. If she didn't like someone she would say it. If she was angry she would tell you in no uncertain terms. If someone corrected her, argued with her, or whispered in front of her she would become very angry and react accordingly. It was more than most of her friends could handle and, understandably, they withdrew.

17
•

I DIDN'T PLAN TO BE
YOUR MOTHER

There is a natural order in family relationships. The grandparents come first, then the parents and then the children. Parents take care of the children. Children receive and parents give. With illness and dementia that is not always how it goes. The natural order of a family system becomes disrupted.

It is common when a parent or a spouse suffers from dementia that the roles in the relationship change. A daughter may find herself parenting the mother, and a husband may step into a paternal role or a carer's role. This can become very disheartening for the family. On the one hand we want our loved one to keep their role in the family as mother, wife or father, husband, and on the other hand we have to take that role away for the safety and dignity of that person.

Mary knows this experience well. 'Before Alzheimer's visited my house, dementia was a term for old people that lived far away. Something everyone gets if they live long enough. But Alzheimer's . . . became part of my family and took my dad . . . away, one event at a time. Have you ever wondered what goes through the mind of a toddler as they mature and grow? Taking care of a person with dementia is like playing the record back-wards. Every day, the things that are so common soon lose meaning. A spoon, how to put on a shirt, disliking a favourite food. Temper tantrums, diapers. Those are the things that I think of when I think of dementia. Life in reverse.'

There is a thin line between supporting our parents and taking over for them. Throughout this time often I felt that I was taking over and was burdened by the responsibility. Another feeling, one that I had not experienced since I was a wild teen-ager in the late 1960s and 1970s, began to creep in. I felt I was being deceptive. Every time I spoke to someone about Lily I felt disloyal. I knew that the old Lily, the one I had grown up with, would have been furious with me for 'hanging our dirty washing out' for all to see. She believed that what happened in the family stayed in the family. I never heard her complain about family to any of her friends. Even when we were children, at our most rebellious, she would tell her friends how wonderful we were and boasted how we always told her everything.

Lily shadowed Lionel all day. She became suspicious that Lionel, Donna and I were plotting things behind her back. It became impossible to speak to Lionel about how he was feeling in front of Lily. He dared not say he was struggling because Lily would become angry with him. She never let him answer the home phone. Sometimes I rang up and could hear the television blaring in the background. It being five o'clock in the evening, I knew they were sitting together on the couch sipping wine and eating crackers and cheese, but she would tell me he was working and hang up.

I tried calling his mobile but before I could ask him how he was, he would give Lily the phone to extinguish any irrational fears she might have had and, just as I asked to speak to Lionel, she would hang up.

L+L

It was Friday afternoon and I could hear Lily and Lionel's footsteps coming up our steps. Lily was on the verge of tears and Lionel looked pale and haggard. Neither of them had any strength to tell us what had happened. Later that night, Oren took Lionel outside on the veranda to have a talk. Almost immediately Lily began looking for him. 'Where's Lionel? Where's Lionel?' she repeated.

I gently took her hand and told her he was outside talking to Oren. She began to walk to the door, mumbling that she had to see him. I told her that Oren had a problem and needed to talk to Lionel and suddenly that seemed to make sense. 'Let's do the washing up together,' I suggested.

We walked over to the sink and I began to recite a poem Lily knew by heart. Music and poetry could distract Lily and transform most moments of despair into moments of joy. Music has the power to reach the emotions of most people with dementia. For Lily it became an alternative way of communicating. The capacity to comprehend music is commonly retained even when language abilities have been lost.

Singing or reciting a poem with Lily was a way to converse with her without confronting her in the areas that no longer functioned well.

Suzy is the kitchen maid,
Who lives across the way,
And from my kitchen window
I see her every day,
Washing dishes!
But the strangest thing to me,
Is the way she's always smiling
As if she likes washing dishes!

Truthfully, I can't say if this poem really exists or if Lily once made it up. It was one of her favourite poems and she loved reciting it. In a flash Lionel was forgotten and we were washing dishes and repeating the poem over and over, adding more intonation, more drama and more incredulity to the words, 'as if she *likes* washing dishes!' By the time the dishes were done Lily had forgotten she was looking for Lionel. Lionel, on the other hand, was by now sitting on the sofa, his rounded shoulders barely able to hold the weight of his head.

That night Oren told me, 'He says he sometimes hopes he won't wake up in the morning.' I didn't know what to say. Together we lay in silence until we fell asleep.

The next day I phoned the Alzheimer's Association, who told me to call the Aged Care Assessment Team.

Trying unsuccessfully to sound calm, I found instead that my voice came out an octave higher than usual. The receptionist informed me no one could see us for a few weeks as the geriatrician was overseas at a conference. I burst into tears. 'But my dad cannot cope any longer. He just can't cope.' The voice at the other end spoke slowly and assured me they would do everything they could. I sobbed out a tear-drenched thank you. My unrestrained gratitude left the person on the other end of the phone speechless.

And then I rang Lionel. He listened, thanked me and hung up. I sat for a long time replaying his 'thank you' over and over. Then I walked outside and stood in the warm afternoon sun and shivered into a cloudy, cold and uncertain future.

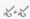

Two professionals from the Aged Care Assessment Team actually came to see Lily the very next week. I told her they were friends of mine and they wanted to meet her. She seemed happy with that. It had taken countless surreptitious phone calls to Lionel's mobile phone to arrange this meeting we had all been postponing for years. Lily responded so well we were amazed. With some regret, we realised help had always been available, had we been able to ask.

18

•

WHISPERING BEHIND HER BACK

As more people became involved in supporting Lionel, he and I found we needed to talk more often together. We needed to share information, plan dates to meet with the geriatrician and community workers. I wanted to stay connected and to let him know he was not alone but the more I contacted Lionel the more creative Lily became in preventing it. She knew something was happening to her and I am sure she knew things were going on behind her back.

Occasionally she would ask Lionel what was happening to her and he answered that it was nothing, everything was fine, and she would let the conversation drop. I can't imagine how confusing that must have been for her. But she knew all was not well and she became suspicious and fearful of every phone call. She began to occasionally forget who I was and thought I was romantically involved with her Lionel and she would tell me to leave her home. If I tried to explain that I was 'Sharon' she would become furious and yell at me, 'Well, *Sharon*, goodbye, good luck and carry on,' and walk me to the door. She became suspicious of her nieces calling, imagining they were strangers pursuing her husband. She refused to let anyone speak to Lionel on the phone.

Phone calls were now strategically planned to avoid Lily answering the phone. Lionel and I tried to send each other text messages and plan a conversation. If she did answer, however, I knew she would tell me Lionel was not there and she would hang up.

There was no reasoning with Lily anymore. She was incapable of changing because the disease itself had created the paranoia. So I gave up reasoning and began to validate her. Whatever she said, I tried to find a way to go with her, not against her.

When the needs of a person with dementia are not met they will often react with aggression or anger. These needs can be physical, emotional or spiritual. Understanding these needs requires calm and compassion with a dash of creativity.

The next time the phone rang I happened to be standing next to Lily as she picked it up. Lily spoke abruptly. 'Hello. Yes? Carole? No, Lionel is not here. I don't know when he'll be back. He's at work. Goodbye.'

She banged the phone down and turned to me, furiously claiming Carole was trying to take Lionel away from her. Speaking in the same tone as Lily, I said, 'Some people just can't get a good man like you did, Mama.'

Lily softened a little and nodded her head. I decided to take the conversation even further and added, 'Well, let's not tell Lionel she rang. Let's keep it a secret from him.' As Lily had probably never kept a secret from Lionel in her life she covered her mouth in shock and said, 'Oh, I can't do that. I have to tell him.'

'Mummy, you are such a good wife.' Lily walked into Lionel's office and told him someone had just phoned. She had no idea who it was but the anger had gone. I helped her out and whispered in her ear, 'It was Carole.'

Lily replied, 'Oh yes, Carole called. We must have them for dinner soon.'

Lionel nodded and agreed to have them for dinner soon.

'You have a good man there,' I told Lily.

'I know,' she said, melting into his arms.

19

•

DO YOU REMEMBER ONE SEPTEMBER AFTERNOON?

The day Lionel collapsed, Lily looked a million dollars. Lionel had spent all morning choosing her clothes and making sure her shoes and handbag matched. He had lovingly put on her makeup, pencilling on her eyebrows into a perfect arch. He took the glass pyramid bottle of Trésor perfume and sprayed her wrists, dabbing a little behind her ears.

It was the Day of Atonement (Yom Kippur), an important Jewish holy day, and the synagogue was full. They found their seats, front row centre, the same seats they had occupied for fifty-five years.

As Lionel silently slid between his seat and the cedar partition in front of him, a hand grabbed the back of his collar and held on tight. Someone had seen him slump and had reached out, just before he crumpled to the floor.

Lily stood very still, hand over her mouth as people jumped the seats and tried to revive him. When the ambulance arrived she stepped up into the passenger seat with surprising ease, gripped her handbag to her chest and looked straight ahead. Lionel was in the back, oxygen mask covering his nose and mouth.

Both my sister and I received the call around twelve noon, 'Your father has collapsed and has been taken to hospital.' Our two cars pulled into the hospital grounds like synchronised swimmers.

'Mummy! Here we are.' We hugged her and told her Lionel would be all right. She forced herself to nod. She could not be left alone. She had long forgotten how to boil water, let alone cook. Lionel had preserved her dignity by making sure she was washed and dressed and well fed. He took her shopping. He suggested they go to restaurants and he drove them to the movies every week. He made arrangements to see friends and he prepared all the food when they had visitors. As Lionel lay in hospital awaiting surgery and an unknown future, Lily's future was equally uncertain.

20
·

WHERE'S LIONEL?

Donna moved in the first week to look after Lily. She told me, 'I left home at seventeen and haven't spent a night in my parents' home since. More than thirty years later I am back, with my little overnight bag, eyeing the sad, single bed in the bedroom across the hall from my parents' room, churning between uneasiness and a strong desire to mother my mother well and lovingly.'

Lily asked repeatedly where Lionel was, and each time we told her he was in hospital she became anxious. Eventually we told her he had gone to work or was away on a conference. Lily knew about work and conferences. The anxiety subsided.

Donna has always been good with Lily. 'I know how to make her laugh. We sing and dance. Usually I visited both my parents, and then took Mum out for an hour or so, to give Dad a break and to enjoy her on my own. I love being with her— there are not so many places that I can laugh and sing and dance out in public with legitimacy.'

Yet as good as she was, living with her was different. 'This wasn't an hour walking along the street, and singing those marching songs that Mum must have learnt during wartime. This was a solid week of time together.'

During that week Donna discovered the full extent to which dementia was affecting our mother. 'I heard how much she talked to herself. She talked to herself incessantly. Dad had told me how her talking drove him mad, but I had not heard it before. During that week she often got angry with me, and would walk out of the front door, or into the garden, sulking and cross. I learnt that the way to bring her back was to go out and tell her how much I loved her. Sometimes she would tell me she loved me too and it would be forgotten. Sometimes she would soften, reluctantly, and I would see an opening to sing one of her favourite songs and she would forget about being angry. Sometimes nothing worked and I would have to watch through the glass door, ensuring her safety and keeping my distance for a while.

'At night I brought our dinner into bed. I lay a towel over the sheets and we would pretend we were visiting the Queen—Mum had a thing about the queen. After only a few mouthfuls, she would put the food aside and snuggle down beside me. She is a little woman, my mama. Lying in bed beside her, I felt the same love as a mother for a child. She would open her eyes and see me there watching her, and we would smile at each other, and she felt reassured and settled into sleep quickly and deeply.'

On the day of our father's surgery Lily was like a record with a deep crack in it. No matter how we distracted her she asked, 'Where's Lionel?' again and again. Donna and I took turns taking her for walks and cups of coffee. Having completely forgotten she had just had coffee, she happily accepted our invitation every time.

When that no longer worked she paced the corridor. She greeted every nurse or patient as if they were guests in her home. 'You must come and visit again soon,' she told everyone she passed. Eventually Lionel was wheeled back into his room.

Lily took his hand, held it and for the next hour muttered words that were impossible to understand.

Over the next few days Lionel pondered on what to do once he returned home. Could he continue to care for Lily in the way he had been doing or was it time to move her into a residential care facility? The day before he was discharged, after many conversations with family and friends Lionel sighed, 'I can't do this alone anymore.'

'Do you mean full-time care?' I asked.

He nodded in silence.

How quickly the wheels begin to turn once a decision has been made. A few phone calls later it was all arranged. In ten days Lionel would take Lily to her new home, a Residential Care Unit for people with dementia.

Lionel came home and began to recuperate. Lily forgot he had ever been in hospital. She forgot he couldn't care for himself. She forgot he could not care for her. She became frustrated, disorientated, confused and angry. I spent that week caring for them both.

Every night I would fall onto the single bed in the guest room exhausted. Sleep came in fits and starts. Lily was due to move into the Residential Care Unit in two days and I worried how she would settle. I worried how Lionel would manage without her. I worried that their life as they knew it was about to end. I worried whether we were doing the right thing. I worried that I was taking control of my parents' life.

Donna was not convinced this was the right way to go. She wanted to create a roster system where professional carers would come in and she and I would take it in turns to support Dad in caring for Mum. She felt it was our moral duty to care for our own mother. I didn't agree with her. I felt Mum would be better off in a home. The tension between us was painful and added to the heartbreak we were both experiencing. Dad's mind was made up, though. I remember drifting off in the early hours of the morning recalling the sound of Lionel's voice saying, 'I can't do this alone anymore.' Somehow, it gave me the strength to do what I had to do.

21
·

THE LAST NIGHT

Holding my breath, I closed the door behind us. The blinding light of the early morning sun brought tears to my eyes. Suddenly, walking felt like wading knee high in mud. It was eight o'clock on Sunday morning and I felt the dull weight of guilt hang from my shoulders like a smelly old shawl.

Lily had always had a long and passionate relationship with hairdressers. As far back as I can remember she would go to the hairdressers every single day. Once a week she would have a wash and blow-dry, and every other day she would jump into the car, drive the ten minutes to Alexander or Charles or Philippe or whoever was the hairdresser of the moment and let them comb her hair up.

A few months after Lily began to show signs of dementia she became impatient with everyone and was unable to sit for long periods of time. Sitting still was unbearable. She needed to move, all the time. I could never have imagined my immaculately coiffed, beautifully made-up, extroverted socialite mother losing all interest in her appearance. Trips to the hairdressers became a battle between Lionel and Lily. Lionel made the appointment, and when the day arrived, Lily would refuse to go. Lionel tried to convince her by telling her she would be so beautiful. He told her he would stay with her. He assured her it would not even cost anything. Nothing worked until he changed tactics. 'Okay, let's go down to the mall and do some shopping.'

With Lily having completely forgotten where they were going, they arrived at the hairdressers and Lily greeted Edward with her usual effusive warmth. Lionel walked away, tired, exhausted and for a moment relieved to have succeeded once more in keeping things more or less normal.

Lily had known Rose for almost thirty years. As the dementia advanced, Lily's old friends had withdrawn—except for Rose. Rose was the only friend who knew how to communicate with her. Lionel and I planned for Rose to take Lily out for the day, a trip that included a visit to the hairdresser's. It was all part of a bigger plan. A secret plan. A heavy, guilt-ridden plan to make the final arrangements to move Lily into the Residential Care Unit, where she would be cared for in a way that Lionel could no longer provide. After his heart attack he had surrendered to the unimaginable.

That day, my mother would leave the world she had always known. We were taking her away. Away from her kitchen and her bed, her tissue-stuffed handbags, her overflowing drawers, her beloved garden where she and Lionel sat every evening, toasting each other with glasses of wine. Away from her hidden love letters, her photos, her wardrobes, her bathroom and her precious jewellery. Away from her suburb and the neighbours she had grown to love. Away from the strangers she had greeted warmly for years on her daily trips to the shopping mall, away from all that was familiar to her. And worst of all, away from her lover, her rock, her knight in shining armour, her husband of fifty-five years.

I walked into her bedroom and began to slowly take clothes out of her wardrobe, clothes that I felt I had no right to even touch. I chose her most beautiful clothes to pack, the ones she stopped wearing a long time ago, preferring the same t-shirt and track pants, sometimes for days at a time. Lifting out a favourite garment, I held it to my face and breathed in the heavy scent of her perfume. I reverently placed makeup foundation, an eye pencil, blush, toothbrush and toothpaste in a small vanity bag and suddenly stopped. I shuddered as I realised that I couldn't put her toothbrush in the bag yet. She would need it for tomorrow.

Oh my God. What am I doing? She isn't dead and I am behaving as if she is. My cheeks burned with shame. I was taking my mother away tomorrow. I was betraying her. While placing the bag of clothes into the boot of my car, I suddenly remembered I hadn't packed her nighties, and ran, like a burglar, back to her room to retrieve them. My head began to spin and I felt sick to the stomach, just as the door bell rang and there she was. Home.

Her hair newly coloured, streaked and cut, her makeup applied perfectly, she looked beautiful. I wanted to tell her, *Mummy, I have packed your clothes and perfume and makeup and handbags into the car. I am trying to do this well. To do this right.* But the voice in my head was screaming, *You traitor. You betrayer. How can you do this to your own mother?*

We sat in silence and ate Thai takeaway. Lionel was unusually quiet, and every once in a while I heard a choking sound. I couldn't bear to look at them. To my relief, they went to bed early.

I sat in the television room and although the TV was on I saw and heard nothing. All I heard was a mantra that refused to give me a moment's peace: *This is the last time they will sleep together.* I curled up on the couch and finally, after holding on all day, I let myself cry. I sobbed into the couch cushion. I poured out my grief and despair and helplessness for all the years that brought us to this place. I cried my pain and sorrow that my parents lay in their marriage bed for the last time. I imagined my father's anguish as he lay there, feeling the soft curling of my mother's legs around his legs, smelling her sweet familiar fragrance, and kissing and holding her in their bed together. He knew all this and carried it alone. I dragged myself into the guest room, lay in bed and prayed. I fell into a restless sleep, dreading the following morning.

I heard her before I saw her. A tiny, gorgeously coiffed woman crept into my room and looked to see who was in the bed.

'Hi, Mama. It's me, Sharon.'

Her quizzical look exploded into a huge smile and she ran into my arms.

'Let's go and have a shower, darling,' I said, and she enthusiastically agreed. I dressed her in a new black t-shirt that I had bought for her the previous day, black pants and a pearl necklace. I put on her makeup and fixed her hair, though it seemed not to have moved all night. Lionel made a pot of tea. On anniversaries, birthdays and Mother's Day, he used to carry a tray with a rose and a gift, along with one slice of toast and a pot of tea, and serve her in bed. But today we met in the kitchen and drank the tea together in a strained lightheartedness.

'We are going out now together,' I announced, wishing Lionel would say something, but he appeared unable to utter a word. Lily began the ritual of announcing she had lost her handbag and we began to look around the house, under chairs, pillows, in the fridge. We found it in the fridge. I took her bag out and handed it to her.

I don't want her to cry, to scream, to beg us not to do this. I can't do it.

I am terrified.

'Come, Mama. We are going to the car.'

'Where's Lionel?' she asked.

'I'm right here.'

It was time.

Holding my breath, I closed the door behind us. The blinding brightness of the early morning sun brought tears to my eyes. Walking felt like wading knee-high in mud. It was eight o'clock on Sunday morning, yet I felt the dull weight of guilt hang from my shoulders like a smelly old shawl. With my mother's tiny, soft hand in mine, I led her away from her home for the very last time.

'Mummy, I want to tell you where we are going today.'

22
·

WHEN I LOST YOU
(ONCE, TWICE, THREE TIMES . . .)

Dementia took memory, language, and independence away from Lily. We grieved the losses as they came. Sometimes loss felt like the sea lapping up against the surface of the sand, sucking a few loose grains back into the sea, and other times it felt like great insatiable waves gulped huge chunks into the ocean. We watched her forget her grandchildren, her friends and her place in her world. As dementia progressed we lost her over and over again.

The day before Lily moved into the Residential Care Unit, Oren and I took a few of Lily's precious paintings off her lounge room wall and hung them in her new room. We carefully hung her clothes in the tiny wardrobe and placed her makeup and creams in the sterile white bathroom cabinet. I placed photos of all our family around the room and sprayed the air with her favourite perfume. I looked around the room that was about to become Lily's home, mentally checking I had not forgotten anything. I missed the irony completely.

Lily sat in the back of the car and as I was driving I could not look at her as I spoke.

'Lionel cannot take care of you by himself any longer, Mama.' She looked out the car window and said nothing. 'You are going to a new home, where beautiful people will care for you and we will come and see you every day.'

She nodded, deep in her own world, unreachable in her thoughts.

The staff insisted we not stay too long. Donna, Lionel, Oren and I drove to the beach and sat together. As we walked towards a bench to sit and contemplate the enormity of the day, Lionel said, 'I feel so empty-handed.' He literally could not recall the last time he had walked outside without holding Lily's hand.

23

·

I'M JUST MAD ABOUT LIONEL AND HE'S JUST MAD ABOUT ME

Sunday mornings were special when I was a child. We were allowed to turn on the television as early as we wanted, as long as we did not disturb Lily and Lionel. Even though on weekdays we were forbidden to help ourselves to food without asking, we were encouraged to get our own breakfast on Sundays.

For years we had no idea why we were given these privileges on Sunday mornings. Donna and I accepted that was the way it was. Later, we discovered what Lily and Lionel were doing behind their closed door and we secretly longed to return to our original innocence. They came out of their room overly interested in what we were watching on television. How do you describe the Road Runner or Tom and Jerry when you are six years old? And anyway, they rarely waited to hear, being too distracted by each other. Lily and Lionel were often distracted by each other.

As I grew up, Lily would recall the moment she fell in love with Lionel. It coincided with her very first orgasm. This story, told with starry eyes that made me deeply uncomfortable, became embellished over the years. It was her wedding night.

She was nervous and he was her knight in shining armour; gallant, chivalrous and experienced. She had no idea what to do and surrendered to Lionel's skilled touch. The orgasm arrived unexpectedly, the story goes, and she felt such overwhelming love and adoration for her new husband that all she wanted to do was make love with him all night.

Although social events brought out Lily's flirtatious side, when asked whether he minded, Lionel always replied, 'Not at all. I'm the one she comes home with.'

Notwithstanding the onset of prostate cancer in his seventies, held at bay with a medication that listed impotency as its most common side effect, Lily and Lionel loved going to bed. They cuddled and whispered and held each other in a loving embrace until sleep took over. As dementia progressed, bedtime came earlier and earlier. A combination of red wine and ever-lengthening silences carried them to the only place where all confusion, pain and sorrow dissolved as they melted into each other's arms. The heart and body knew what to do, even if the mind did not.

Making love was of such great importance and pleasure for Lily and Lionel that the notion of it coming to an end was unthinkable. But it did.

A single bed, set starkly against the mauve painted wall, brought their physical delight to an abrupt end. As I looked around the room that was to become my mother's new home, a voice in my head was screaming, *But where will Lionel sleep? She has never slept in a single bed for fifty-five years!*

Deeply disturbed, Donna and I called a meeting with the staff. 'Our parents like to sleep together. They cuddle and hold each other every night. Where can Lionel sleep if he wants to be with her? Where can they be intimate?'

'We have "do not disturb" signs you can request from the nurses station.'

'But can't we put a double bed in there? It's only thing that still brings them joy.'

'We realise it is not one hundred per cent satisfactory but for the time being there are no double beds in the Residential Care Unit.'

As the months passed and my parents spent their nights far from each other, their daytime cuddles became limited to greetings and farewells. Lily had always been the physically demonstrative half of the partnership but now she could not initiate what they both used to love so much. In fact, when Lionel informed her at the end of his visit that it was time for him to go, Lily sometimes withheld her hug in protest. Lionel would try to hug her and Lily in a flash of anger would walk away, declaring, 'I'll never forgive you. Never!'

Of course the next day, when Lionel returned, Lily would throw herself into his arms and hold on for dear life. As passionate as that was, it did not have the timeless ease of their long, tender hugs of bygone days.

The first few weeks in the Residential Care Unit were almost unbearable. Lily was not settling down in the manner we had been told she would. She paced the corridors tirelessly. She called out for Lionel incessantly and looked for him in every room.

I did not know how to help her. Feelings bubbled up and leaked into my days at unexpected moments. I could be standing in a shop and a wave of grief would rise up and without warning I would burst into tears. I woke up night after night dreaming of Lily alone in her room. I still could not believe we had actually placed her into a Residential Care Unit. I felt tired and sad most days and didn't want to see friends or talk on the phone to anyone. I stopped writing. I stopped reading. I missed her.

I did not know what to say to friends. I thought, *Maybe I could say I feel like my mother has died*, but the words would not come out. My feelings didn't match the reality. My mother had not died. Emotionally, however, I felt there had been a death in the family yet there was no body to bury. No gathering of friends to share sweet memories and bid my mother farewell. No public acknowledgment of her life and who she was. When I learnt that this feeling had a name—disenfranchised grief—I was relieved. Labels can sometimes be so comforting.

Disenfranchised grief is the grief people feel when a loss cannot be openly acknowledged, publicly mourned, or socially supported.

24

•

WHAT'S LOVE GOT TO
DO WITH IT?

He never actually said it, but he wrote it in poetry on scraps of paper, usually found lying beside the phone. Every anniversary, birthday and Mother's day, Lionel wrote a verse or a rhyme to Lily, declaring his undying love.

When the sweltering heat of summer rose up and crinkled the air, turning the steep tar road outside our home into a blue shimmering haze, I begged Lionel to let me sit in the back of his Ford Zephyr as he made his annual pilgrimage to the corner newsagency. Exchanging a few dollars for a small, black, pocket diary, he tenderly carried it home and awaited inspiration. In the early hours of the morning, I heard him tiptoeing down the creaky, dark hall to his study. As Lily continued dreaming, Lionel reverently opened the diary and, holding his red and black fountain pen, would begin his annual tryst with last year's joys and sorrows. Then he would spill out his optimistic dreams and hopes and blessings for the year to come.

When the grand poem was complete, he presented the diary to Lily and she, without fail, wept with joy as she read his ode to the one he loved. She would then put her new diary in her handbag and for the next few weeks show the poem to everyone she met.

Lily loved her diaries, perhaps even more than she loved Lionel, sometimes. She would read and re-read them, taking pleasure in her tears that smudged the ink and left the words a little harder to read every year. She would often take her diary out of her bag and read to Donna and me the poem that was carrying her through another year. By the time Lily moved into the Residential Care Unit there were over fifty diaries lying in a cardboard box on the top shelf of her wardrobe.

Heavy with grief, the day after Lily had moved into the Residential Care Unit, Lionel was going through her things when he came across another box. It had a faded image of a small-waisted woman wearing a pastel sun dress, long white gloves, and a pale blue hat. It contained every card and note he had ever written to her. Lionel and I sat on the bed she would never sleep in again, and read together for hours. He had not only penned his love and appreciation, but as the notes revealed, he often tried to reassure her that she was truly loved. He apologised for perceived grievances she appeared to be holding against him and reminded her that when all was said and done, their love would carry them through all of life's rugged undulations. Letter after letter declared his love and gratitude. Letter after letter begged her to trust that all would be well. Letter after letter implored her to believe him and to remember how much she was loved.

As I sat on the bed with Lionel, I wondered what could have caused her to feel so insecure. 'Why didn't she trust that you loved her unconditionally?' I asked.

'I don't know. I just had to keep on telling her. She worried about her financial security. She was always concerned about us not having enough money to live the way she wanted.'

'But she never wanted for anything,' I insisted.

'She rarely bought herself anything. Everything she had, I bought for her.'

I looked at Lionel. 'Never? What about when you went overseas?'

He said that although he encouraged her to go shopping with the other wives, she never bought anything for herself. 'Later, we would go out together and I would buy her something. I always loved to see her wearing a beautiful dress or a special piece of jewellery.'

'And when you were not travelling, did she buy things for herself then?'

He shook his head. 'I don't know. I really don't know why she never wanted to buy herself anything.'

He was still holding some of the cards he had written to her. 'Daddy, did Mum ever write you birthday or anniversary cards?'

He scratched his head and looked past me. 'Actually, she never wrote me a note in all the years we were married.'

25
·

I DON'T THINK I LOVE
HER ANYMORE

Lily, once adept at beginning and carrying on a conversation, was now limited in her ability to verbally express herself. Unlike Donna and I, who were comfortable singing songs and playing with Lily, such ways of relating did not come naturally to Lionel. Where once she could chat with him about anything and he would add snippets of his own ideas, he now no longer knew how to engage her. Where once he had managed most of her physical needs, the main tasks were now attended to by the nurses in the Residential Care Unit. He no longer knew how to be Lily's husband.

The texture of love changes as our loved one is no longer able to share the moments of intimacy that once defined the relationship.

They were sitting opposite each other, two empty coffee cups between them. Lionel was massaging hand cream into Lily's thin, age-spot covered arms, and Lily was staring at the movement of the trees outside. They were not talking; in fact it seemed in some strange way that they were unaware of each other. I broke their reverie and sat down beside them.

Lionel was upset. He was unscrewing a tube of moisturising cream. 'I don't know. I ask them to put moisturiser on her every day but I don't think they're doing it. Her legs are terrible.' Lily started to pull up her pants to show me her legs. 'No, no, no, leave your legs alone,' Lionel said a little too loudly.

Lily began to scratch her leg. It had three or four squamous cell carcinomas that were bothering her. 'Stop scratching your leg!' Lionel admonished her. Lily stopped and looked at me, like a three-year-old child who had just been chastised.

'Mama, let's go for a walk in the garden.'

Lionel stood up. 'I have to go home. I've got some work waiting for me and I need to do it before tomorrow. Bye, sweetheart. See you tomorrow.' Lionel bent over to kiss her on the cheek.

'I'm coming with you. I'm going home, too.' Lily was shocked.

'No, sweetheart, I've got to go and do some work. I'll be back tomorrow.'

He scratched his head, in the way he always did when he was upset, and walked towards the exit.

I took Lily's arm and we began to walk towards the garden. I started to sing, 'Do You Remember One September Afternoon?' and Lily joined in.

That night I called Lionel to check if he was all right. 'I don't know. I just don't know.' He sounded exhausted. 'What don't you know, Daddy?'

'I don't know if I love your mother anymore.'

I wanted to say, *Yes you do! Of course you do. You'll never stop loving her. Remember all the letters and the cards? Remember the diaries?* But not a word came out.

'She's not the girl I married.'

No, Daddy, she's not the girl you married.

'I don't think I'll go tomorrow. I need a little break.'

It took every ounce of my strength to hold back the tidal wave building up in my throat and behind my eyes. 'It's okay, Daddy, I'm going tomorrow anyway. It's really okay to take a day off for yourself once in a while.'

Silence.

'Good night, Daddy. Sleep well.'

'Good night, sweetheart.'

I placed the phone in its cradle and wept. And I know, I just know, Lionel did the same.

26

•

I WANT A KISS TOO

There is a photo of a young and beautiful Lily on the door of her room. Lionel stuck it there one day, thinking it would help Lily find her room. Lily sees her and tries to talk to her. 'Hello, my darling,' she says to the photo. She waits and then looks at me. 'She never talks to me. We were old friends. I've known her for years and years.' She turns around, bends forward and kisses the young lips that never speak.

I put out my arms and whisper, 'Mama, I want a kiss too.' She puts her arms around me and we hug. I never want to let her go.

27

NOW DON'T YOU WORRY, I'M JUST DYING

Every visit was traumatic at first. Every time I saw her she grabbed me and held on as if she was drowning. She cried out to God in gratitude that I had arrived. We stood holding each other, exposed, vulnerable and always observed by the staff. Privacy was gone. Our laughter, our singing, our tears were all seen and heard and witnessed. Staff would come over and tell me what Lily had done that day in front of her, and I wanted to tell them to stop. I wanted to yell, *Go away. Don't tell me all this. Don't talk about my mother as if she isn't here. Who cares? Lily doesn't remember, so why tell me? You are confusing her.*

All I wanted to do was hold Lily and protect her from a world she had no way of understanding. Lily, who never wanted her guests at home to stay too long and reluctantly agreed to have the occasional grandchild sleep over, was now expected to live with thirty people with dementia. This group of individuals, many of whom would not have been friends in the outside world, were now all expected to live together.

Lily didn't like the other residents. Some of them frightened her, including one in particular who had lost the ability to show any emotion on her face and who would follow Lily everywhere she went. Countless times a day Lily would look nervously over her shoulder and, realising she was being followed, yell out, 'Go away! Leave me alone.'

It was bad enough to leave your home, your husband and your world to live in an institution but to live with someone who terrifies you—that was more than I could bear for Lily.

One morning I visited Lily and she hobbled towards me. Hobbled! Lily never hobbled but today she could barely walk and her head appeared too heavy for her small frame to hold up. Her hands were shaking as she inched herself towards me.

'Mama, what's the matter?' I was shocked and frightened.

'It's time,' her voice quivered. 'I'm going to die here. It's over.'

'Are you sick?'

'Yes, very sick.' And then she looked at me and said, 'Now don't you worry. You will be all right. I'm dying.'

As shocking as that was to hear, it was all the more appalling since Lily had never, in her life, talked about death. She had avoided going to her father's funeral. She had seen no point in travelling halfway across the world to attend her brother's funeral and when her sister died she refused to have her name included in the death notice in the newspaper. I have sometimes wondered whether Lily's marrying a doctor in some illogical way convinced her of her own immortality.

I recalled an incident from my childhood. Lily adored her mother and when she died Lily lay lifeless in bed for a whole day. I had been forbidden to enter her room. 'Is she going to die?' I asked the maid. Taking no heed of my youthful anxiety, she mumbled something that sounded like, 'Yes dear, you be a good girl and go outside and play.' I remember feeling the spiny prickles of cold fear jabbing my whole body all at once as I walked outside to wait for my mother to die.

The next day, however, Lily got up, dressed in a fitted navy-blue silk dress with white polka dots and went to play cards with her friends. When Lionel came home from work she was especially overjoyed and clung to him with renewed vigour, smudging red lipstick all over his cheek.

Standing now with my arms around Lily, I felt that familiar prickle. I was losing Lily, again. 'Mama, it is going to be all right.' I walked into the social worker's office. We needed to talk.

That night sleep was pushed away by obsessive, recalcitrant thoughts. What went wrong? What was the matter with Lily? Although I had always believed everything happened for a reason, I found it impossible to even imagine what that could be. Finally, in the early hours of the morning with my brain in painful overload, I fell asleep.

I called Donna at 5 am and we decided we would arrange an emergency meeting as soon as possible. Although we drove to the Residential Care Unit separately, as usual Donna and I arrived together. Brenda, the clinical director and Yvonne, the social worker, looked at each other as if each hoping the other would begin.

'We have been talking,' began Brenda, 'and we think we may have missed some important information about Lily. We were wondering whether your mother ever drank alcohol?'

'What?'

'Did she drink alcohol?'

'Well, she loved her evening drink of wine with Lionel.'

'How often did they do that?'

Donna and I looked at each other. 'Nearly every day.'

'How much would you say she drank?'

'Oh, not much. One or two glasses. Maybe more, very occasionally.'

'Well, actually,' Donna added, 'sometimes they did drink a few more glasses and once or twice Lily fell asleep before she ate dinner.' We smiled at each other uncomfortably and I quickly added, 'But not often.'

Brenda and Yvonne looked at each other. 'Did she drink every day or was it occasionally?'

I felt defensive and angry. 'She drank a glass of wine every day.' I was thinking to myself, *This is an investigation, not a conversation.* 'She wasn't an alcoholic if that's what you are thinking.'

Brenda continued in her calm, professional manner. 'Did she ever ask to have a drink early?'

'Yes, but Lionel wouldn't give it to her.' I was breathing fast and hoped no one could hear my heart beating. 'He was quite clear it was their evening drink.'

I felt I was in a courtroom. My face became hot and flushed and I began to feel dizzy. I needed some air but the next question left me unable to stand up.

'How long would you say Lily had been drinking a glass or two of wine?'

I thought about all the dinner parties. The charity balls and cocktail parties. The days where Lily would not drink a glass or two were the exception.

Donna and I looked at each other and I whispered, 'A long time.'

'Well, it sounds as if Lily was dependent on her daily drink of wine and when she arrived in the Residential Care Unit, all that stopped. It is possible—actually it is probable—that she is in alcohol withdrawal. Even three glasses of wine a day can create a dependency and suddenly stopping can cause her to go into withdrawal.'

I wanted to tell them they were wrong. It was impossible.

'How long will it take before she is feeling better?'

'We don't know. Perhaps a few more weeks. We just have to wait.'

I looked at Lily. Curled up on the chair, pale, shaking, oblivious to the conversation she had just heard. 'Mama, you are going to be all right soon. You are going to get better. Donna and I are here. We'll help you.'

Lily smiled and cuddled into Donna. 'It's going to be all right. Don't you worry,' she said as she patted Donna's hand.

While dementia caused Lily to feel confused, ashamed and disoriented, alcohol left her feeling relaxed, sociable and light-hearted. More like the old Lily. Although a couple of glasses of wine every day would not normally be considered a serious alcohol problem, alcohol can have detrimental effects on the progression of dementia. It has the potential to exacerbate vascular dementia and the effects can vary significantly, depending on the height and weight of the person.

The day Lily and Lionel were married Lily weighed 97 pounds or 44 kilograms. After giving birth to each child she returned to her pre-birth weight, give or take a kilo. Being so slight certainly had a significant impact on the effect of alcohol on her system. One or two glasses of wine on average is unlikely to have a detrimental effect on the majority of people; however, in those early days, when Lily realised she might be losing her grip on controlling her life, she increased her consumption of alcohol.

This is not unusual. Some people find that by increasing the amount of alcohol they drink, they feel—at least temporarily—that they are more able to deal with the frightening changes in their memory and consequently their life.

It is important to say here that alcohol abuse can lead to several forms of dementia, but, according to Lindsay Farrer, head of the genetics program at the Boston University of Medicine and founder of MIRAGE,[15] it does not seem to cause Alzheimer's disease. In a MIRAGE cross-sectional study, Dr Farrer and a team of researchers assessed retrospective alcohol use among Alzheimer's patients and their cognitively normal siblings.[16] They observed a protective effect of a moderate alcohol intake (ie, consumption within USDA recommended guidelines of one drink per day for women and two drinks per day for men). The potential protective effect, which is small to start with, may be related to the anti-oxidants contained in some alcohol beverages such as red wine.

Dr Farrer adds, however, that there are still many important questions about the way the existing research information is gathered and what is moderate drinking for one person may be excessive for another.

28
.

NURSE, NURSE!

Settling in to residential care always requires a period of transition and generally takes anything from three weeks to eight weeks but for Lily it took about three months. The staff at the Residential Care Unit learnt how to relate to her, always smiling when they spoke. Lily could tell in a flash who was being sincere and who was patronising her and she let them know in no uncertain terms. Jean worked in the kitchen and she recognised that if she asked Lily to help her, Lily became stronger and happier by the day. Jean genuinely liked Lily and Lily could tell. Jean would dab a bit of makeup on her in the morning and take her to the main kitchen, chatting all the time like they were friends. Lily needed to feel useful and Jean not only saw that but found different things for Lily to do around the Residential Care Unit.

Some of the staff learnt the songs Lily loved to sing and I was deeply moved when I arrived one day to see a beautiful Filipina nurse singing 'I Belong to Glasgow' with Lily. The nurses invited her to go for walks in the garden and as there was often music playing she loved to dance with Lionel when he visited. The pain of separation from Lionel began to ease.

Then, just as she was feeling more settled, Lily began to complain about her legs. Scarred from her many falls and flaking with dry skin no matter how much moisturiser was massaged into them, Lily's legs became the centre of her life. She scratched them with such vigour that her socks were often stiff with dried blood. No matter how we tried to distract her, nothing could ease the incessant itch or sooth the continual pain of the small lumps that were growing on her legs.

29
·

THE COPPERTONE KIDS

Being 'brown as a berry' signified good health in my family forty-five years ago. Most weekends, Lily and Lionel would take us to the same beach where we swam in the warm water of the sheltered cove as they chatted with friends, smoked cigarettes and slathered baby oil on their smooth, youthful bodies.

Without fail, we came home sunburnt at the beginning of every summer season, and were assured that once we had peeled we would be fine for the rest of the summer. Indeed, we were 'as brown as berries' by the time summer had ended. I remember the pain of my red-streaked little body as it cringed under the torrent of warm water washing away the sand and salt of our day at the beach.

'You won't even remember this tomorrow,' Lily would tell me as I winced.

L+L

The pain in Lily's legs had become unbearable. Those poor legs. They were so sun-damaged that the dermatologist burnt off new sun-spots every month. Before she went into the Residential Care

Unit she had fallen a number of times and seriously skinned her shins. The combination of sun damage and repeated falls had resulted in a dozen or so squamous cell carcinomas on her lower legs. They were excruciatingly painful and Lily would not allow anyone to touch them.

The only way to relieve her pain was to remove the carcinomas under general anaesthetic. An appointment was made for the following week. We were instructed to arrive at the hospital at 7 am to be admitted. By 8.30 am we were in her hospital room waiting to go into theatre. By 12.30 pm we were still waiting. By 2.30 pm still waiting. Lily walked and walked up and down the corridor. She was a caged animal without food or water. The doctor had placed her at the end of his list.

We all began to wither as hour bled into interminable hour. We told Lily why she was in hospital and she asked us again and again and again. She yelled at the nurses who walked into her room. She curled into Lionel's shoulder like a shrivelled autumn leaf.

Three-thirty . . . still waiting. By 4.30, we were parched and exhausted. At 5 pm two orderlies wheeled an oil-thirsty gurney into her room and asked Lily to climb up. She panicked. 'Where am I going? I don't want to go.' The orderlies started to explain the whole procedure to Lily, but she started to scream, 'No! No! NOOOOO!'

Softly, I whispered in her ear that it would be all right. 'We are with you, darling. Don't be frightened.' She climbed up onto the gurney and sat upright. Lionel and I walked beside Lily until we reached the thick plastic curtain dividing us from the operating theatre and then we were told we could go no further.

'Please,' I begged, 'she has Alzheimer's. Please let my father come in, just till she is asleep.'

'No, impossible.' They were immovable.

They wheeled her away. Lionel and I held onto each other as she screamed and screamed, 'I want my daddy, I want my daddy! I want my daddy!' Boiling hot tears stung my eyes and streaked salty rivulets down my cheeks. *She won't remember this tomorrow. But I will.*

We wouldn't ignore a five-year-old child begging for their mother or father as they are being wheeled into surgery so why do we do it to our loved ones who have regressed in age through dementia? Although these patients may physically look like adults, dementia winds back the emotional and intellectual clock and they cannot understand what is happening. In addition, for all of us, hospital can be a confronting place. For an elderly person with dementia it can be absolutely petrifying.

In the past twelve months Lily has been admitted to hospital twice. On both occasions hospital staff lacked the specific skills to know how to speak to her or how to console her. On both occasions she became so terrified she screamed and cried and fought with both doctors and nurses, believing she was fighting for her life. She was held down, spoken to very loudly, and given long complicated explanations about what they wanted to do to her without her understanding a word.

It would be wonderful if hospital staff were better informed about how to help patients with dementia. If a patient with dementia comes into hospital, it would help if staff were to find out their level of understanding of language. Dementia causes a loss of language, both in expression and in understanding. There is no point explaining a procedure if all the words mean nothing and result in creating more anxiety for the patient.

If someone had told Lily, 'You will be all right. I am here. There is nothing to worry about,' she would have relaxed. Short sentences. There is no point in asking someone with dementia questions like, 'What is your birthday' and 'Why are you here in hospital?' They don't know and you will increase their anxiety. Ask their carer instead.

Touch speaks louder than words. Stroke their forehead. Hold their hand. Tell them how wonderful they are. Be gentle. Be softly spoken. Be loving. Remember, they don't know who you are or why you are doing certain things to them, and no matter how many times you tell them, they will not remember. Sing, hum and smile a lot. Give them a soft doll to hold when you inject them. I mean it. Have soft dolls in every orthopaedic ward because it is usually full of older people and some will have dementia. Give them something delicious to eat. A sweet, a chocolate, a cupcake. Sing a lullaby. And finally, if all else fails, whisper, 'I love you, Lily' (or Jack or Mary or Paul) into their ear. What have you got to lose?

30
·
LOOKING FOR LIONEL

Lily paced the corridors, asking the same question, over and over.

'Where is Lionel? When is he coming?' She stopped the kitchen staff on the way to the dining room to ask them about Lionel. She looked in every room, in every bathroom, in every cupboard. The staff responded as they had been advised.

'Lionel is at work. He is seeing patients and will be here soon.'

'Lionel just called and he will be here as soon as he leaves work.'

'Lionel was called out on an emergency and will be here soon.'

Before she had dementia, Lily loved to know Lionel was at work. He was the breadwinner and it was right that he provided for her. In fact, one of her favourite sayings used to be, 'You marry a man for better or worse, but never for lunch.' Now, for a minute or two after being told that he was at work, she calmed down. Then she would forget, and ask again.

On this particular day Lily was agitated, and kept up her frantic questioning, asking everyone, 'Where is Lionel? . . . Where is Lionel? . . . Where is Lionel?'

Bernie, a new resident who had a predilection for kissing the female residents with Casanova passion, was sitting on a chair with his head in his hands, shaking it from side to side. Shirley, the head nurse, walked up and asked him whether he was all right.

'Should, should I . . .' he tried to get the words out. 'Should I be looking for Lionel too?'

By this time, everyone had joined in the search. The entire Residential Care Unit was galvanised into looking for Lionel. Even those residents who spent most of their days staring into their own private worlds were now pushing their walkers around the unit in an earnest search for Lionel.

And then he walked in. Shirley was busy calming Bernie so she didn't see him. In fact, no one noticed him at first. Suddenly, Lily looked over toward the door and screamed, 'LIONEL!!!! THERE'S LIONEL!' Everyone began to cheer. They called out, 'Lionel! Lionel! There's Lionel,' and the whole unit became united in Lily's joy and jubilation. Tea and coffee arrived—as it always does, every afternoon—and small squares of apple cake were passed around. Celebration was in the air. Lionel had arrived!

31
·

RAINY-DAY FRIENDS

As weeks passed Lily became stronger. She made a friend, and together they walked into all the rooms and up and down the halls. Lily and Clara chatted and although I didn't know what they were saying they seemed to understand each other. When Lionel arrived he kissed Lily hello and Clara would expect a kiss too. I began to look forward to seeing Lily. Especially on Fridays.

The Residential Care Unit was built next door to an existing kindergarten. Every Friday the children arrive at 11.30 am to give a concert to the residents and pass around the morning tea. Sometimes the residents sing and dance with them. It is the best day of the week.

This Friday it was pouring with rain and I had wasted twenty minutes searching for my umbrella. Giving up, I walked out into the rain, opened the car door and saw it on the seat. It took over an hour to drive to the Residential Care Unit and I walked in just as the children were marching up the hall singing, 'See how I'm marching, marching, marching, see how I'm marching, just like this.'

Lily was nowhere to be seen. She was not in her room or Clara's. I asked the staff on duty. But no one could find her.

I heard them before I saw them. At the end of the corridor
Lily and Clara were walking out of the storeroom with their
bags full of towels, cotton wool, terry-towelling bibs and packets
of sanitary pads. They appeared very busy.

'Mummy!' I held my arms wide open and walked towards
her.

She looked at Clara and then back at me.

Clara said, 'Hello, dear.'

My arms slowly slid down to my sides.

'Hi guys. How are you?'

'Is it still raining?' Clara asked.

'Is it still raining?' my mother echoed.

'Yes, it's still raining.'

'We have to go home now, don't we, dear,' Lily ignored me
and spoke to Clara.

'Yes, we do. We have to go home.'

Together they linked arms and walked away, back down the
hall. Suddenly Clara stopped.

'Do you have a . . . one of those . . . uh, one of those things . . .
Oh what is it?'

'An umbrella?' I asked.

'Yes, an umbrella.'

'Yes. Actually, I thought I had lost—'

Clara took it and they walked away.

'Bye bye, dear.'

'Uh, bye Mama, bye Clara.'

They began to sing 'Pack Up Your Troubles in Your Old
Kit Bag'.

I stood there and watched them walk away from me. I looked
around for someone, anyone, to share this moment with, but I
was alone. I smiled as I watched them disappear down the hall.
As I walked to my car I realised it had stopped raining.

L+L

After the settling-in period was over Lily began to flourish. She began to connect to individuals in the Residential Care Unit. Her friendship with Clara, however, was as short as it was intense. They spent every day holding hands and walking up and down the corridor, opening doors and helping themselves to anything that caught their eye. But things happen and old memories get tangled up into new relationships and the knot becomes too tight to unravel. One day they had an argument. It was hard to fully understand what happened but I think Clara stood up to Lily and Lily was crushed and reacted with anger. As quickly as it began, Lily and Clara stopped holding hands and went their own ways.

There is a part of me that loved to see my mother mischievous, childlike and happy. I wish they were still friends.

32

·

LEARNING TO SPEAK DEMENTIA

Alana was a furious 99-year-old with a vocabulary that would make a truckie blush. When I said hello to her, she often would tell me to fuck off. One day she yelled at me, 'Where the fuck did you get that shirt?' I fumbled for something to say when she asked me, 'Did you buy it in London?' Without thinking I said yes, London. 'Oh wonderful,' she said. 'I was born in London. I love London.' From then on, every time she said something, I used the word 'London' and she melted.

'It's fucking cold in here.'

'Just like in London,' I replied.

She instantly softened and said, 'Oh! Yes, yes, I was born in London.'

'Get that stupid bloody table out of my way.'

Without a second thought I said, 'It's as crowded here as the London tube.'

She nodded, 'I know. I know. I was born in London.

I replied, 'I love London.'

'Yes, yes, so do I, lovey, so do I.'

There are some important rules about speaking dementia that will help anyone to pick up the language pretty quickly.

Don't ask questions that require short-term memory. For example don't ask 'How was your day?' or 'Where is your handbag?' or 'What did you have for lunch?' or 'What are you doing?' or 'Did your son come to see you today?' Ask simple questions that require a yes or no answer.

Simple observations work well. *It is a beautiful day today. Can you feel the sun on your face? You look lovely in that dress. I brought you an apple and banana. Which one would you like? I hear you have a beautiful son.* Stay in the moment.

Tell them something interesting. *I couldn't resist buying these cup cakes. I went to a good movie last night. The children did very well at school.*

People with dementia are still interested in things that interested them before. So if your friend loved fashion, ask her whether they like the dress you are wearing. If your mum used to cook great chicken soup, ask her whether she fried the onions or put them in raw. If your dad loved politics, tell him about a new policy or ask his opinion.

Lily loved her work. She loved to go to the art gallery or to the dress shop where she worked for many years. She loves me to tell her about those times. And I tell her the same stories over and over. Before she lost her ability to formulate sentences, I would 'kick start' the story by saying, 'You really know how to make any dress look great,' and she would be off and running about the time she used to sell clothes to the rich and famous.

Notice and focus on their remaining skills. Placing the dishes in the dishwasher became too complicated for Lily but when I gave her a large bowl of beans to top and tail she was able to do that and feel useful again. She knew how to fold tea towels and

I would give her a few from the laundry basket. Other times I would pass her a cloth and she would happily wipe down the bench tops. Always keep the activity within their ability.

33

·

LAUGH AND THE WORLD LAUGHS
WITH YOU

A few months before Lily moved into the Residential Care Unit, we were having lunch at Donna's house. It was a warm Sunday afternoon and Lily chatted and charmed everyone and when it was time to go, Lionel and I walked down to the car with her. She held onto my arm and said, 'I haven't seen Donna for ages.' Lionel turned around and replied, 'What do you mean? You just saw her. This is her place.' Embarrassed, confused and frightened, Lily said, 'Oh, I know *that*. I mean, I mean, Sharon. I haven't seen Sharon for ages.' I quickly jumped in and said, 'I haven't seen Sharon for ages either.' She looked at me and I couldn't resist winking at her. Suddenly she burst out laughing and declared, 'You're Sharon!' I nodded and in a loud voice with my hands above my head I said, 'I am!' We began to laugh. We couldn't stop. Eventually we climbed into the car feeling happy. The shame of forgetting was, for the time being, over.

People with dementia are frightened of making a mistake. They often lose their train of thought and cannot find the right word to express themselves. As caregivers we can help by supplying them with the missing word. We can even finish a sentence as long as we know that is the sentence they wanted to say. But for Lily, laughter was the key to moving through difficult moments. Maybe I'm just lucky but I always found Lily to be funny and when I laughed so did she.

Humour is the key to lightheartedness.

Humour exists in every language. No matter how difficult the situation, if there is a modicum of humour the experience is transformed.

Communicating with someone who has dementia is very different from the way we communicate with others. Most of their understanding does not come from what is being said but how we say it. Body language, attitude, eye contact, tone of voice, touch, acknowledgment, warmth and kindness all contribute to good communication.

34

.

I'M SORRY I MAKE YOU CRY

As a child I would often fabricate stories, grand stories about people I knew, sights I'd seen, or things I'd done. When I was no more than seven years old I wandered up to the local high school to watch the 'big' girls sit under the massive Moreton Bay fig tree and sun their freshly shaven legs. I wanted to shave my legs too. I hated being seven. I wanted to wear stockings and gloves. I wanted to laugh and chat with friends. I was not a popular child.

One day my teacher phoned my mother to ask why I was always late to school. Lily, who insisted on driving me the 500 metres to school, feebly replied she had no idea. The investigation began as soon as I returned home. I created a vivid story of a kookaburra talking to me every day and explained to my mother that even though I *wanted* to get to school on time *it* wouldn't let me!

I now call those 'lies' acts of creative inspiration. They were childish attempts to be validated, to be appreciated, to be valued and indeed to avoid being punished. I don't remember the last lie I told my mother as a child, but I can remember the last time I lied to her. It was yesterday.

We went for a walk and as we so often do we began to sing the 1939 Jimmie Davis song, 'You Are My Sunshine'.[17] Although Lily had almost lost the ability to formulate sentences and respond to me verbally, she could still sing the words of old songs she knew long ago. Linking arms we strode down the street and I began by singing, 'You are my sunshine.' Mum responded theatrically, 'My only sunshine.' Back and forth we went, telling each other, 'You'll never know, dear, how much I love you,' until at the end of the song Lily transformed herself into the famous melodramatic French actress Sarah Bernhardt, clasped her hands to her heart and cried out, 'Oh please don't take my sunshine away.'

We laughed and hugged each other. Lily declared, 'We are so wonderful. We have always been like that. We've known each other for years.' I agreed and said 'You are my sunshine' and we began all over again.

Together we had found a way we could communicate with joy again. Through singing the songs she had loved in her youth, one line at a time, first me and then Lily, I had stumbled onto something very important; another bridge to connecting to my mum.

After thirty minutes of this, we walked, still singing, arm in arm, back to the Residential Care Unit. All was quiet. Everyone was sitting at their tables waiting to be served lunch. The atmosphere was a stark contrast to how we were feeling. It was time for me to leave but she held on tight. 'What do you mean? Where are you going?' She looked shocked and frightened. I tried to explain that I had to go home.

'I'm going home with you,' she said as her grip remained firm. I looked around for someone to take over but everyone was occupied with serving lunch. The first lie tumbled out as I told her I had to go home to cook the children their dinner.

'I will cook with you. Don't leave me here.'

The next lie slipped out like an ice cream falling off the cone and splattering onto the ground. 'The shops are about to close and if I don't go we won't have dinner tonight.'

She looked into my eyes and started to let go.

'Really?' As I took her hand and guided her towards her seat, her eyes filled with tears. 'Don't leave me here. Please don't leave me.'

'I'll come straight back, Mama.' I didn't even blink as I told her this third and final lie of the day. She did not want to sit down so I kissed her and walked away. She stood in the middle of the room, waiting for me to come straight back. I lie to my mother every day now.

I want to rationalise the lies. I want to excuse the fabrications and stories as acts of creative inspiration. I want to say that everyone tells little white lies to soothe, appease and calm their loved one who suffers from dementia. What's wrong with that? These lies soften the harsh reality that I am leaving and Lily is not coming with me. All that is true and yet, as I walk away, I know I just lied to my mother, again.

That night, perhaps to ease the guilt and sadness, I wrote a letter to the staff at the Residential Care Unit.

Dear Nursing Staff,
Please find below a few ways to calm Lily when she is upset. These things usually make her smile.

Remember, she loves to sing. Her favourite songs are:
'I Belong to Glasgow'
'Pack Up Your Troubles'
'It's a Long Way to Tipperary' (She says Tickle Mary).
'Do You Remember One September Afternoon?'
'You Are My Sunshine'.
She will calm down when you tell her Lionel is at work.
She loves to be told she is beautiful (but you have to mean it).

She wants to help. Ask her to set the table or pass around the tea and biscuits.

She loves to have makeup on and then be told she looks young.

She needs to walk and enjoys fast walking outside.

She loves to be asked her opinion, especially about fashion or placement of furniture.

She hates to be ignored.

She hates to be patronised.

She loves to be welcomed, acknowledged and appreciated.

She can be stubborn. Please try not to say NO to her.

She is not good with groups. Don't force her to do anything.

She likes to be the centre of attention.

When all else fails, sing her a song—softly, looking in her eyes.

Tell her, 'You are my sunshine.'

Tell her you will make sure everything is all right.

Tell her she's safe.

Please be kind to my mother. She is the only one I've got.

Thank you,
Sharon

35
•
NOT TODAY

After three months of visiting Lily I woke up one morning knowing I just couldn't bear to see her today. It was not that something in particular had happened, but rather the uncertainty of not knowing who or what would greet me on the other side of the locked door. Would Lily be having a good day or a bad one? Would she be glad to see me or fall sobbing into my arms? Would she remember me or had we reached that moment when she wouldn't know who I was?

I felt worn out. Every time I walked into the Residential Care Unit I had to brace myself for the unexpected. As I pushed the security code into the keypad beside the door I would breathe a smile onto my face. As I swung open the door I would whisper a quick prayer that she had not fallen back into the deep despair of those early days. But it was not the thought of arriving that stopped me today. It was leaving. I didn't have the strength to leave her today.

When I kissed her goodbye all the air would leave her and she would deflate like a wizened balloon. She would whisper, 'Okay,' and put her arms around me. She would stand and watch me walk away, my tears falling unrelentingly with every step.

36

·

GUILT

Although logically I knew I was not doing anything wrong by choosing not to visit my mother I needed to reassure myself. I told myself that missing a day here and there was far better than forcing myself to see my mum when I didn't want to. Still the guilt stuck to me like hot, wet tar.

Lorry, one of those I interviewed for this book, still tears up when she remembers the time during an interview when the nurse asked her father if he was still driving a car. He said, 'No, I gave my keys to my daughter.' She asked, 'Why did you give her your keys?' He answered, 'Because I trust her.' Lorry said, 'Those words—"I trust her"—went through me like a gunshot. I was stunned to hear the words and I felt like I was betraying his trust by helping admit him to the unit.'

After placing her mother in the Residential Care Unit, Roberta told me, 'I really feel badly that she is not getting much of what she needs spiritually. This time last year she knew every prayer and every hymn and she even knew the priest's refrains. But I live so far away I can't help her the way I want anymore. She used to love praying and going to church so much.'

People who care for someone with
dementia often talk about feeling guilty,
even when they are reassured by their friends
and family that they are doing a
wonderful job.[18]

Being connected to a loved one with dementia, especially if you are a carer, opens us to a wide range of emotions. Although caring can be very rewarding, it is also hard work and can be extremely stressful. Some of the emotions that arise, such as grief and anger, are healthy responses to challenging circumstances. They can be useful, helping us to move forward. But other emotions, such as guilt, can be destructive, leaving us feeling powerless or 'stuck'.

Carrying around guilt is exhausting. It consumes the energy we need for other tasks. The first step to addressing guilt is to become aware of it. The second step is to work out where these feelings come from. Thirdly, it is important to remember you are not the only person feeling this way and, finally, find ways to both acknowledge yourself and become more forgiving and gentle with yourself.

One of the reasons we feel guilt is that we make mistakes. Everyone makes mistakes and yet surprisingly few of us appreciate how valuable making a mistake can be. We prefer to treat ourselves harshly.

We may feel guilty that we are ashamed or embarrassed by our loved one's behaviour. We may sometimes wish we could pack, leave everything and go away forever. We may fantasise about our loved one being dead. If you have ever had those thoughts, you are not alone.

And finally unresolved feelings from the past is one of the most difficult experiences to face if the person with dementia criticised, dismissed, belittled or even abused you when you were a child.

In the process of writing this book I met a wonderful woman, Lorry. Whilst her father was often very angry, her mother lived with a mental illness called borderline personality disorder. She writes,

Growing up in a severely dysfunctional family I was told what to think, and how to act. Gut reactions were not allowed. Having an opinion was out of the question. Blind acceptance of the powers that be (my parents) was the only way I knew. I did not love him (Dad). I did not like him. I did, oddly enough, feel a sense of connection to his mother whom I never met. She died when he was three years old so I had a very soft place in my heart for my 'baby dad', the child his beautiful young mother left behind when she died of TB. It was the 'baby dad' who came through when Alzheimer's took its toll. People who grow up in dysfunctional families may hold resentment and conflict as they try to sort out how they feel versus how they believe they should feel.

They may feel guilty that they dislike this person even though he seems so helpless now. They may wish they had made more of an effort to heal the wounds of the past before now. We are often tempted to push ourselves too hard in these circumstances in an attempt to compensate for the past. We would be better off seeking help in resolving the feelings from the past so that we can deal with the present situation.

Sometimes it is hard to forgive ourselves for becoming irritated and angry with our loved one. Accepting that we are under considerable stress is the first step to being gentle with ourselves. Remember, chances are that in an hour or two our loved one will probably not remember we lost our temper, and next time we will have an opportunity to respond the way we would have wanted.

After the person dies we may feel ashamed that we are relieved our loved one is now dead. We have probably been grieving for a long time now for the person who is no longer the person we knew, and as dementia progresses, watching our loved one deteriorate day after day is deeply disturbing.

There are many reasons feelings of guilt arise and the best way to deal with them is to talk to someone you trust. Understanding your feelings and taking time to explore them with friends, or a professional, can help you to make the best choices for yourself and your loved one.

37
·

SLOW DOWN,
YOU MOVE TOO FAST

Brad wore a woollen beanie in summer and winter. He looked like a large weather-beaten old fisherman who had seen and heard it all. He spent most of his day sitting on his 'special' chair at the table where he ate his meals, quietly watching everyone and occasionally dozing off.

Lily, sitting behind Brad, was reciting a poem she had learnt in her youth and had never forgotten, 'Lone Dog', by Irene R. Mcleod. Donna and I were clapping, encouraging her to say it again, when Peter, Brad's son, arrived. He walked over to our table and immediately engaged Donna and me in conversation. Brad turned around in slow motion to see his son.

'Brad, would you like to come over here and sit with us?' I asked. With enormous effort Brad stood up. Turning his chair around for him, I motioned him to sit down. Peter helped settle his dad and then continued talking.

Donna is a professional storyteller and teaches children and adults as well as performing at concerts and events all over the world. There was a concert planned for the next night and Peter was excited to share that he, too, would be performing. He spoke very quickly.

'So,areyougoingtobeattheconcerttomorrownightitisgoingto beamazingandIhavebeenaskedtosingasongmedleybeenwondering whattosingandguesswhoelseisgoingtobethere . . .'

In a deep, slow voice Brad said, 'She said lunch is in an hour.' Peter stopped, looked at his father. 'Yes, Dad, lunch is in an hour.'

'SoIwasthinkingofsingingacoupleofoldiesfirstwhatdoyouthink?' he continued his conversation with Donna.

Brad repeated, 'She said lunch is in an hour.'

Lily was becoming agitated. She needed to have our attention and was unable to follow the conversation. She opened her bag and began to heap tissues onto the table, folding and then placing them one on top of the other, as if she was tidying the linen cupboard. Brad repeated, 'She said lunch is coming in an hour' only this time a little louder and with some agitation.

'Dad, it's okay. Lunch is coming.'

'SoanywayIhearyouareperformingatthegatheringnextSaturday . . .'

'She said that lunch is coming in an hour.'

Lily started to mutter words under her breath as she tore the tissues in half and then folded them again. I stood up. 'Mummy, do you want to go now?'

She stood up and looked at Peter and then said loudly, 'I don't like that man.'

'I know, Mama.' Later, as I was leaving I noticed Brad's head had lolled forward. He had fallen asleep. His lunch lay untouched on his table.

L + L

At the 2008 International Conference on Alzheimer's disease, Jeanne Katzman[19] from the University of California presented a paper on the effects of Alzheimer's on family conversation at dinnertime. Thirty families in which one member had recent onset of Alzheimer's participated in her three-year study. Each family had two videotaped dinner conversations which were later transcribed and analysed. The goal was to document ordinary family conversations and to analyse problem areas that arose with Alzheimer's.

Katzman found the responses of healthy family members to words uttered by the family member with Alzheimer's followed certain predictable patterns. When a response was unexpected and disrupted the normal flow of conversation, healthy family members often were observed to continue their talk almost as if the person with Alzheimer's had not spoken. Even though the healthy family members tended to pause—a sign that they had heard the person with Alzheimer's—they did not respond verbally.

This lack of response meant the person with Alzheimer's did not participate in the conversation.

Katzman found many families regularly explained what the person with Alzheimer's was trying to say and indeed often spoke for the person. She found that families with only two members conversed in a greater variety of ways. Responses often took the form of rewording; the healthy speaker suggested what the other wanted to say, expanded upon it, and brought the contribution of the family member with Alzheimer's to a close.

Katzman says, 'Family members often develop assumptions and expectations about their conversational roles and responsibilities. With the onset and progression of Alzheimer's, the person with dementia becomes less able to speak as others have always expected him or her to.' Difficulty in finding the right words was the most noted inability, followed by shortened attention span and/or impaired short-term memory. The individual is no longer able to follow another speaker's retelling of the day's events.

In an attempt to participate in the conversation, the person with dementia may say something that shows confusion or misunderstanding. He may initiate an unrelated topic because he cannot remember what had just been discussed.

Recently I returned from a trip to Japan and went to visit Lily. I told her I had been to Japan. She exclaimed, 'Japan!' and I began to tell her about it when she said, 'And then they come . . . and I . . . thank you very much . . . but I have to go . . . so thank you and goodbye . . .'

The story of Japan melted away and I took her hand and whispered, 'I am home now, Mummy. I love you so much.' She began to cry and we hugged each other. Japan is over, and all that matters is that we are here, right now, together.

38
.
DROPPING DOWN A GEAR

Peter was not a bad son. He simply had not changed gears. He was travelling at the same speed he had always travelled. When a loved one, friend or patient has dementia we are called to drop down a gear or two, and allow ourselves to become still. To wait a few extra moments. It can take time for a smile of welcome or a nod of recognition to occur and if we move too fast we will miss it. Sometimes as dementia progresses responses may take even longer and there will come a time when there is no response. However, the more centred and present we are when we are with our loved one, the more likely they will respond to us even in some small way.

Peter's usual way of behaving may not have been disrespectful when Brad was well, but it became inappropriate as the disease progressed.

Another tip that can make the world of difference is not to argue with your loved one. They are right and you are wrong. No matter what. It's not easy, especially if you still have unresolved issues with your parent. My suggestion is if you can't accept that whatever happened in the past is OVER, then take some time for yourself to heal the past by doing some counselling or personal growth work, otherwise you will never be fully present with your loved one now. I have found that disagreeing with Lily—even when she says something obviously incorrect—results in her becoming irritated, angry and upset. It is not worth it.

There is a man who lives in the Residential Care Unit with my mother and he always wears a suit. He is a good-looking man. I tell him every time I visit how handsome he looks and every time he smiles and walks over and we chat about the weather. He loves to watch the cars coming and going through the window and sometimes I sit with him and say, 'The cars are coming and going.' And he nods and tells me something about the cars. Sometimes I don't understand exactly what he says but I act as if I do. The connection is always a warm and happy time between us.

Speak slowly and use short words and simple sentences. People with dementia not only lose their ability to use language, they lose the ability to understand it too. So listen carefully and repeat whatever you said as many times as necessary.

Be prepared to *hear* the same sentence or the same story over and over and be prepared to *say* the same sentence or story over and over. Short-term memory loss means the person with dementia gets stuck in a loop and can only say what they see right now. Listen with respect. In other words, affirm what you heard them say. Jolene Brackey, author of *Creating Moments of Joy*, says to 'distract rather than react'. Take a bag of peas to shell together, fold the tea towels or give a manicure, sing a favourite song. And if it works, repeat it again and again.

39

·

LOOK AT ME, WALK WITH ME, TALK TO ME

Smile, hug, kiss and show affection. Sensory stimuli are important communicators. Slow down the process and wait. It takes someone with dementia longer to respond to being touched, stroked or kissed.

Speak a little more slowly, make sentences shorter and make eye contact. Look into their eyes and see beyond the condition. This person is a soul and if you take time to really be with them your loving presence is probably enough; verbal communication might not even be needed.

Do not multi-task. Speaking on your cell phone to conduct business or chat with a friend while you are visiting someone with dementia may feel rude or dismissive to them. It could feel like you are saying, 'You are not worth my attention.'

I have said it before but it is so important I want to say it again. Do not argue with a person with dementia. Try not to ask, 'How are you?' It can take you down a road that has no happy ending. When things are not going well they will often get stuck in trying to express themselves. If you are visiting your loved one, tell her that her hair looks wonderful, but only if you mean it. It will bring a little joy into her day. Tell her that you heard she was a wonderful cook. (Only if you did hear that—compliment the person on a skill you know they once took pride in.)

Don't invalidate his or her imagination. Stay with the story and share something simple of your own. If they are upset, hallucinating or delusional, as sometimes happens with a person with dementia, don't argue but when feasible, redirect them to a photograph, a video, a song or a story.

Play music from his or her time period, not yours! And keep it simple and cosy. Too many visitors can easily overwhelm or overstimulate and upset the routine.

Manage your own personal stress levels and take time for yourself. People with dementia are often extremely sensitive and will absorb your stress.

Just as you would not speak over a friend or a child, speaking over a person with dementia effectively excludes them from the conversation. Include your loved one in the conversation as much as possible.

40
·
THE KEY IS VALIDATION

As the lift door opened, I heard Lily screaming, 'Leave me alone! Leave me alone!' Pushing her walker past slower residents, she flew into the lounge and saw me. Lifting her arms above her head, she praised God. I put my arms around her and she began to sob into my shoulder.

'Mama, you are very upset,' I said. She nodded. 'Did something bad happen just now?' She nodded, and tried to tell me what happened but words without connection tumbled out. I listened, nodded and eventually said, 'Sometimes it's not easy, is it?' She hugged me tighter and repeated, 'Yes, yes, yes'. With my arm around her tiny bony body, we walked to her room.

As soon as we sat on her bed, Lily started to rummage in her bag. It was exploding with paper hand towels. She collected a few every time she walked down the corridor and put them in her bag. She took out a bundle and gestured for me to take them. 'I would like you to have this. They are mine but I want you to have them.' Not only was I touched by her obvious generosity but I was amazed at her clarity of speech. I took the bundle of paper towels and told her I would treasure the gift. She beamed.

Later, I arrived home and took the bundle of paper towels from my handbag. I put them inside the box that holds all my old letters and imagined someone finding the box in fifty years and wondering why, amongst the birthday, anniversary and love letters, there lay a pile of crumpled paper towels.

People with dementia develop many different kinds of behaviours. Executive Director of the Validation Training Institute in Cleveland, Ohio, Naomi Feil, realised many behaviours can be understood as an attempt to complete and resolve unfinished life issues. Feil calls this final phase Resolution. 'In Resolution, very old people try to tie up the emotional loose threads of their lives before death. In very old age, they face tasks they should have faced years earlier.'[20]

Although Lily had settled into life at the Residential Care Unit, she tried to avoid interaction with the other residents unless she initiated it herself. Occasionally, Lily would say, 'Look at them. They're all crazy.' She would roll her eyes and get up and try to get away from the other residents. She distanced herself from these people who reminded her of the one thing she had most feared. Going mad. When I was a child, my mother would often scream at me that I was driving her crazy. In a fit of fury she would threaten to brain me. I didn't know what that meant but I could hear the sheer panic in her voice. She could not handle being questioned, challenged or corrected. If I dared to say anything that contradicted her, she would explode with rage. Could her father have gone crazy from the brain tumour just before he died? Perhaps. And maybe the way her father died had remained unresolved for Lily all her life.

Don't ask your loved one if they remember you. In fact, don't ask them, 'Do you remember . . .' anything. That is a 'never ask that question' question! Recently I heard a nurse ask a resident with advanced dementia if she remembered her. It is not relevant, and in any case a 'yes' does not mean that they do remember.

Ironically, it is one of the most common question friends and family ask their loved ones. Lily found a wonderful way to answer. She started to sing, 'Do You Remember One September Afternoon?' She sang this song a hundred times a day. The truth, however, was that she would soothe herself by singing the song because the question would unsettle and disturb her.

Lily was afraid of losing control and now in her old age, to keep herself together, she hoarded. Paper towels, tissues, scraps of paper, combs and lipsticks all crammed into a handbag that was never off her shoulder. Understanding this has helped me to know her better. Normalising her emotions, validating her feelings always calms her down and leaves her feeling at peace again.

Many years ago when our children were young, I would read them a story by Mem Fox. It was a book about a little boy whose name is the full title of the book, *Wilfrid Gordon McDonald Partridge*.[21] He lived next door to a nursing home and he knew everyone who lived there. One day he overheard his parents talking about Miss Nancy. They said she had lost her memory and Wilfrid Gordon McDonald Partridge set out to find it for her. The book touched me deeply. One day Wilfrid Gordon McDonald Partridge brought her a basket of his own treasures to show Miss Nancy and one by one they triggered in her a treasured memory.

Although losing one's memory is a significant part of dementia, objects can still trigger emotions, and even stories. Outside each person's room in the Residential Care Unit is a memory box, intended to hold some treasures from that person's life. The idea was also to help them find their own room. Strolling down the corridor is a walk down memory lane. Some of the memory boxes are full of photos, tiny vases, porcelain objects and spiritual memorabilia. Recently I saw a pair of Sabbath candles in a woman's memory box. I thought of her lighting those candles every Friday night for sixty years or more. One man has some war medals in his memory box and nothing else. I wondered what stories those medals hold.

Lily's memory box holds a few photos and two tiny teddies dressed in wedding clothes. It was a gift given to Lily and Lionel on their fiftieth wedding anniversary and she loved it. Recently, I pointed out the teddies in the memory box and told her the story: a beautiful girl called Lily had met a handsome doctor over fifty-six years ago. I told her that they fell in love and never wanted to leave each other. I told her that after only ten short weeks they were married . . . I told her Lionel had loved her more than anyone in the whole world and had taken her to wonderful places—Italy, France, Greece and even China. She listened, cried, nodded and hugged me. She whispered, 'I remember. I remember.' Whether she did or whether she didn't doesn't matter anymore. What matters is that the memory box reminds me of the stories I can tell my mother. Stories she loves to hear again and again.

41
COMING TO OUR SENSES

I scooped up a large glob of hand lotion and warmed it between my hands. Lily stretched out her thin, dry arm and slowly, so, so slowly, I began the sacred ritual. First I hold her palm in mine and gently lay my hand on hers. Without moving, I let my palms whisper their greeting. She closed her eyes. That was the sign to begin, and as if to the slow rhythmic beat of an ancient drum, I massaged the lotion into her hand. Every finger absorbed my full attention. I stopped thinking and my hands took over, moving up her forearms, softening the parched spots that thirstily soaked up the moisture. She smiled. There was no need to speak a single word. Mother and daughter present and peaceful. Our minds still. Sitting in stillness together.

Even if your loved one doesn't recognise you or can't communicate verbally, there are many ways to show reassurance and love. People with dementia can still experience the world through their senses.

For me touch is the most effective of the senses. It is the first thing we do with a newborn. We touch its soft velvety skin and we feel engulfed in love.

42

•

MEETING AGAIN
FOR THE FIRST TIME

It was lunchtime when I arrived and Lily, sitting having lunch, did not notice me. I saw Eleanor perched on the narrow seat of her walker. I had chatted with her many times. She was rocking back and forward, saying, 'I want to see my son. When is he coming? Where is he?' She repeated this over and over. I hesitated. Usually when I visited Lily she became upset if I spent too long chatting with anyone else. But she had not seen me arrive and so I walked over to Eleanor. She looked up at me and asked 'Where is my son?'

I introduced myself, adding that I knew her son. He and I had met a few times at the Residential Care Unit and I thought it would be a point of contact. A nurse walked over—a new nurse whom I had never met before. 'She is always just asking for her son. Don't worry about her. He'll come later.'

I looked at Eleanor and she was pleading, 'Where's my son? I want to talk to him. I want to go home.' I sat down next to her and began to talk to her. I told her that I knew she missed her son. 'Yes. Yes. I want to go home. Please take me home.'

Sitting close, I repeated, 'You want to go home and see your son.'

She began to nod and reached out to hold my hand. 'Yes. I want to go home. I don't have the key. He has my key.'

'Eleanor,' I asked, 'tell me, what does your house look like?' She began to tell me in detail.

'It's very big, many people. I had a big kitchen. Yellow flowers.'

'How beautiful,' I smiled. 'I love yellow flowers.'

'Yes, yes, and the children came home.' Eleanor was talking softly now.

'How many children do you have, Eleanor?'

She was looking directly into my eyes.

'Three.' We were connecting deeply and I told her that I have three boys too. She nodded.

'But it was a lot of work,' I added. 'All that shopping and cooking and driving them around.'

She nodded in agreement, 'Too much work. I don't do it anymore. They are grown up. I don't want to work now. I'm too old. I want to rest.'

'Eleanor,' I said, meaning every word, 'you deserve to have a rest. You did a wonderful job with your boys.' She smiled and reached out her other hand and asked me, 'What is your name?'

'I'm Sharon.'

'I'm Eleanor.'

We gently shook hands and for a few minutes neither of us wanted to let go.

L + L

As the French adage goes, the heart has reasons that reason itself cannot know. The pathway to the soul is the heart, not logic or reason: words or gestures can be the vehicles. When we connect to an old person's reality, rather than reason with them logically, they feel validated and acknowledged.

Get into their world and look around.

Whatever they say is right, even if you know it isn't. Join them wherever they are. Get into their world. That is the only world where you will once again be in positive contact with your loved one. If you join them in their current 'world' or time, wherever that may be, you will be much more likely to find moments of real joy together again. Value what remains as much or more than grieving what is lost.

Lily loved working in the kitchen and giving her the opportunity to rinse the dishes brought her immediate pleasure. Eleanor wanted to see her son, but she also wanted to go home. Rather than telling her logically that this place was her home now, I asked her about her home. By talking to her about her sons and her home she was able to tell me that she was glad they had grown up and that she no longer had to do all that work anymore. She became more peaceful.

43

·

GET OFF MY CHAIR!

'You're sitting in my chair! That's my chair. Get up. It's MY chair. MINE. GET UP! GET UP!' Lily looked up from our conversation, startled to hear Sybil shout at her. She shouted back, 'Go away! Go home. You're crazy. Go away!'

The argument escalated. I turned to Lily and whispered in her ear. 'It's too noisy here. Let's go to your room and we can put makeup on.' She nodded, so I turned to Sybil. 'Sybil, this *is* your chair. You are right. This is your chair. Would you like to sit down?'

'Yes. Yes, I want to sit down on MY chair.'

I put my arms around Lily and stroked her shoulder gently and she stood up. We began to walk to her room, leaving Sybil to sit on the chair that clearly represented something very important for her.

L+L

Very old people who have not prepared for the physical and psychological blows of ageing often use symbols to express their human needs. Sybil, for example, was using the chair to express some inner need. She was in a stage called mal-orientation, where people fear change.[22] They have generally led productive lives but have failed to complete certain life tasks. They need to express their emotions that have been bottled up throughout their lives. They have not learnt to face pain, anger, frustration, shame, guilt. Throughout life, they have denied painful emotions. In very old age, the denial worsens. They blame others for their own failures. Speak to the emotion behind the loss of words.

When we tune into their inner world, we begin to understand that a retreat into personal history is a survival strategy, not mental illness. We are then better prepared to listen with empathy rather than frustration when they step away from reality.

44

·

YOUR MOTHER
IS A VIOLENT WOMAN

Fifty years later I can still remember the ringing in my ears. If it hadn't hurt so much I think the sound would have fascinated me. The funny thing is I never turned around and ran before her beautifully manicured hand made contact with the side of my face. I could taste her rage long before I felt it. Sometimes it only took a look, a sniff, a cough or a shrug of the shoulders to ignite her fury. I never learnt to keep quiet at those times. The words tumbled, and the slap spun my head around before I could take a breath.

So when Jane, the registered nurse, loudly informed me, 'Your mother is a very violent woman,' I can truthfully say I was not shocked. I was embarrassed. I was taken aback. I was even apologetic, but I was not shocked.

There were days in the Residential Care Unit when Lily was disturbed, upset, frustrated and angry. These were the days she wore her tight black leggings, pink striped t-shirt and her short black jacket. Her overfull brown handbag hung heavily across her thin body and she paced the corridor, up and down, up and down. At the end of the corridor she pulled the handle of the locked door and tried to force it open. She said something under her breath, turned around and furiously strode up towards the lounge. She looked around at the residents in utter disgust and proceeded to march back down towards the locked door again. But today was different. She was sitting very quietly when I arrived.

She hardly noticed me. I found Jane and said, 'Mum seems very quiet. Has she been given some medication?'

Jane almost spat out the words, 'Your mother actually injured one of the residents today. One of the residents said something to her and she just lashed out. Your mother is a very violent woman.' For a moment I couldn't speak.

I looked at Lily and suddenly remembered she had been wearing those black tights and the pink t-shirt two days ago. Squeezing out the words, I asked Jane whether Lily had been given a shower today. She replied that she didn't know. 'I wasn't here this morning.' Feeling my own anger rising up, I asked her if she would mind looking in her chart, please.

The chart revealed that she had not been showered for the last two days. She was scheduled to have a shower at 5.30 am every morning. What was happening? I asked. Jane looked at her chart and then remembered something. The nurse who usually helped shower Lily had been sent to another section of the unit two days ago.

Jane added, 'Your mother really got on well with her, too.'

I wondered how it must be for Mum, living in this strange environment, making one close connection with someone and then suddenly not seeing her anymore. Another person taken away. Enough to make her want to lash out at anyone, I imagine. 'Can you get her back?' I asked. To her credit, Jane promised to do her best.

I sat down beside Lily and hugged her, cheek to cheek. Something suddenly reminded me of the old rebel that used to live inside my mother. I whispered, 'Let's get the fuck out of this place.' Her face lit up immediately and she repeated, 'Let's get the fuck out of this place.' As we marched toward the locked door she told me, 'You know that door, it never opens.' I pressed the code. 5, 4, 3, 2, OK. The door opened and Lily squeezed my arm in joy. 'I love you so much. I just love you.'

'I love you too, Mama.'

Just as a child in kindergarten will lash out when he is frustrated or frightened so too will an adult with dementia. In the early to middle stages of dementia knowing something is wrong is terrifying. Fear then leads to suspicion, anger, frustration, tears and depression.

When a close relationship with a nurse is interrupted or the routine has been changed the person may feel unsafe and become anxious and aggressive. They cannot explain this and so carers need skills to either interpret the problem or divert the energy away from the problem.

Jolene Brackey, author of *Creating Moments of Joy*, suggests that there are two magic words that seem to calm down most upsets: I'M SORRY.

I'm sorry. I didn't know.

I'm sorry. I did not mean to hurt you.

I'm sorry. That should not have happened.

I'm sorry. You are right. (Even if you did nothing wrong, say it anyway. It works.)

Acknowledge your loved one sincerely and often.

I often thank my mother for being the mother she was. I learnt so much from her. She was optimistic and positive. She could organise a gathering with unlimited style and grace. She modelled behaviour that offered me choices. In some ways I chose not to be like my mother. That too was a gift.

When Lily lashed out it was her way of saying, *stop, enough, leave me alone, back off, I'm frightened.* Over time as dementia progressed, Lily no longer remembered that she no longer remembered. The things that used to upset her, the locked door, the change of staff, the occasional remark made by another resident, affected her less.

A few weeks later, I arrived intending to take her out for lunch and jokingly whispered, 'Let's get out of this place.' She held my arm tight, shook her head and said, 'Not today.' I looked around the room to find a couple of chairs so we could sit down inside, and it occurred to me I was also looking for the lost rebel.

45
•

I WONDER WHO'S KISSING
HER NOW?

When I first saw Ora Mae I couldn't believe my eyes. She was kicking up her heels as the piano accordionist belted out 'Hava Nagila', the Hebrew song of celebration. Swinging her dress from side to side, she danced with uninhibited enthusiasm. She was a new resident and she was ninety-eight years old. The second time I saw Ora Mae she was sitting next to Henry, and they were holding hands. Suddenly, she leaned over and began to kiss him. Not just a peck on the cheek. No. They were kissing with a passionate fervour. A nurse walked over and gently tried to distract them.

'Ora Mae. Ahem, Ora Mae can you help me carry this to the kitchen? Hello, Ora Mae!'

No response except that Henry was now getting more and more excited and all the residents had one or both hands over their own mouths.

'Henry, HENRY! Let's go out for a walk, Henry. Can you hear me, Henry?'

Everyone in the unit was riveted to the spectacle.

'Ora Mae. ORA MAE! You have to stop. Henry is married.'

Ora Mae looked up in surprise and asked, 'I'm married?'

'No, darling. Henry is married.'

Again she asked, 'Henry and I are married?'

'No, you are not married but Henry is married and his wife will be very upset.'

'I'm not married?'

'No, Ora Mae. You are not married to Henry. Henry is married to Lorraine.'

She looked into the nurse's eyes and said, 'Oh, shut up.' By now Ora Mae was becoming very frustrated and she turned to Henry, put her arms around his neck and began kissing him again.

One of the nurses told Henry that his wife was coming to see him in a minute. Another nurse asked Ora Mae if she would like a 'nice cup of tea'. Henry was helped to his feet and distracted and slowly, reluctantly, Ora Mae followed the nurse to the kitchen.

People with dementia often lose inhibitions and make advances to others. They may undress or fondle themselves in public. Sometimes they may mistake another person for their partner. Their need for closeness is very important. Closeness and touching is a natural part of people's lives, including people with dementia. Sexual needs do not stop because someone is old or has dementia. Unless we take the time to talk to the person with dementia whose behaviour is overtly sexual we will never understand the underlying need that they are trying to express. For many people with dementia, sexuality is bound up with feelings of loneliness, past rejections, abandonment and even unrequited love.

Ora Mae was regarded as a very difficult resident. She was angry and often aggressive except when she was dancing or being overtly sexual. The response of staff was to try to control her behaviour. She was given medication to calm her down. One day I asked a nurse where she was and was told she had been moved to the high-care section of the home.

46
·

CHERISHED MOMENTS

Lily always knows my face but she no longer knows I am her daughter. One day I was putting some makeup on her and she looked in the mirror. She looked at her face and became distressed. She pulled her cheeks up and back, trying to smooth out the wrinkles. I realised that although she still recognised herself, she definitely did not remember how old she was. Curious to know how old Lily thought she was, I asked her. 'Twenty-three,' she responded immediately.

'You are beautiful, Mummy. Do you know why I call you Mummy?'

She looked at me and tears filled her eyes and she said, 'Because you are my mummy.'

I just said, 'Yes. You are my mummy.'

It is no longer important whether Lily knows who I am, only that I love her.

Toilet-paper letter

I visited Lily late in the afternoon, intending to spend a couple of hours with her before going to a lecture in the evening. I saw her walking down the hall with one of the diversional thera-pists, Howard. I waved but she didn't recognise me, until we were face to face. She said, 'I've had enough now,' and I asked her if she wanted to rest. She nodded, said goodbye, and walked away from me.

'It's okay,' I told Howard, and added, 'I'll go out to the kiosk and have a cup of coffee.'

About fifteen minutes later, Howard walked over to me with Lily. She was sad and teary. Howard mentioned that she been calling for me. It sometimes happened that sadness overtook Lily and she became enveloped in melancholy. She began to search in her handbag. She took out a pen and a long piece of toilet paper. I smoothed the toilet paper out on the table and Lily wrote me a letter without any prompting.

Dear Sharon,
I am Lily. Lionel and Sharon love too. We together and Donna.
Love,
Mama

She gave it to me and I read it aloud. Moved to tears, I turned the page over and wrote her a letter.

Dear Mama,
I am Sharon. Lionel and Donna love you so much. I love you too and together we are a family.
Do you want a cup of coffee?
Love,
Sharon

As always, she cried from the first word but when she reached the end she began to laugh. Folding the toilet paper into a tiny scrunched-up ball, she managed to stuff it into her handbag. 'I will keep it forever.' She probably will.

Tissues and toilet paper became her money and when we went out together, she very lovingly gave me a sheet or two of toilet paper to pay for our coffees. I always took it and said thank you, assuring her that next time I would pick up the bill.

The gracious bow

It was Saturday and Lily looked well. 'Look! There are some quoits over there,' I said to Lily, pointing to the chair. Lily walked over and picked up the soft black rubber rings. She held them but did not know what to do with them. 'Can I go first?' I asked and took one of the rings from her. I threw and missed. I threw again. By now Lily had got the idea and she threw and missed too. She looked at me. 'Throw another one. Go on, throw again,' I told her. She threw and missed again but this time she didn't look at me. She prepared herself, took aim and threw. The black ring spun around the wooden post and landed, clunk. Lily screamed in delight.

One of the residents, who was sleeping on the couch, jumped at the shrill sound of her scream. Lily threw again. It landed perfectly on the ring. We whooped and jumped with joy like ten-year-olds. A few residents and a nurse wandered down the hall to see what the noise was about. Lily threw again. The ring hit the top of the wooden stick and stopped for a split second before sliding down and resting on the base. We screamed and clapped and laughed and so did the residents who had gathered around to watch. Again she threw. Again it hit its mark. Lily was beaming with joy. She looked over at everyone clapping and made a little bow.

He is she and she is he

'Hi, Mama.'

'There are some people here I don't like. I don't like him,' said Lily pointing to a woman walking slowly past her in the opposite direction.

'I think that is a woman,' I suggested softly.

'No! It's a man.'

'Oh! Well, I like his skirt.'

Lily looked at the skirt and burst into laughter. I'm not sure if it was because she realised it was a woman or if the sight of a man wearing a skirt amused her.

The gift of Lily

When I arrived, Lily was sitting on a chair tossing a large plastic ball to the nurse in the centre. Actually, it looked more like she wanted to knock the nurse over, given the ferocity of her throw. As soon as she saw me she jumped up, ran towards me, threw her head back and thanked God over and over that I had arrived.

This was a very different Lily to the one I had been visiting lately; in fact it was a very different Lily to the one I had known all my life. The only time I remember Lily in direct contact with God was when she prayed, 'God help you if you don't do what you are told.' The need to be recognised or remembered has long passed. Now my mother falls in love with me every day. No past pain and no future plans. To be cherished and loved anew by Lily every day is a gift.

Fifty-five years!

'How would you like to celebrate your anniversary?' I asked Lionel. Lily had been in the Residential Care Unit for only two weeks. He shrugged in the way he usually did when he was unsure of what to do. We had been advised not to take Lily out for a few weeks. Let her settle down first, they said. We spoke to the social worker and told her about the approaching event. 'We could create an anniversary dinner for you right here,' the social worker suggested.

Two days before the big day, Lionel and I rummaged through Lily's wardrobe at home and found a slightly stained, pink pants-suit. The nurse promised to have it washed and ready for the big day.

Donna, Lionel and Oren arrived together. Lionel walked in wearing a crisply ironed pale blue shirt, silvery-blue tie and navy jacket. His style never wavered with his advancing years. The nursing staff had taken Lily to the hairdressers during the day and she had one of those teased bouffant styles of the 1970s. When she saw us, she literally ran into Lionel's arms smudging pink lipstick on his lips.

The staff had placed a centrepiece of fresh flowers on the table. Lifting small glasses of purple grape juice, we made a grand toast. 'To Mummy and Daddy. Lily and Lionel.' Lily took a sip of the grape juice and said it was delicious and then stood up to make a speech. 'This is the best night of my life. I will never forget it.'

Lionel meticulously arranged the photos of the night into an album. He lovingly worked on it for hours. Over the next few months Lily cried every time she saw the album. 'We have been married for fifty-five years,' Lionel would tell her. 'Fifty . . . five . . . years!' she would respond with amazement.

To this day we still tell her the story of the night she will never forget.

47

·

SINGING ME SOFTLY

Lily and I slowly made our way down the hall towards the sound of the violin. It was one of *those* days. Lily was fed up with everyone. She said, 'Goodbye, good luck and carry on,' to everyone who sat beside her and jumped up from her seat only to remember she was still in pain from her leg surgery and sit back down again in despair.

We walked past Pat and Sam. I had a soft spot for Pat. She was the first person to phone Lionel the day Lily moved in to the Residential Care Unit. She knew it would be a day he needed support and she was right. I would never forget her kindness. Pat once told me that the day the doctor told Sam, 'You have Alzheimer's,' Sam stopped talking altogether. He never said another word. That was nine years ago. She never left his side until the day she collapsed with exhaustion and reluctantly agreed the time had come to place Sam into special care.

The sound of the violin was like a delicate fragrance that wafted down the corridor and guided us towards the music room. Intimately holding the instrument under her chin, Nicola the music therapist was oblivious to our arrival. She was from Armenia and music ran in her veins.

Edelweiss, edelweiss . . . Lily and I linked arms and began to sway from side to side. The strains of the violin filled the room and Pat began to sing in her well-trained soprano voice. Everyone joined in.

I turned to smile but noticed Pat crying.

'What's wrong?' I whispered. She shook her head as if to say, *Not now.*

I persisted. 'Are you okay?' She leaned over and said, 'They just told me Sam is being moved to a higher care unit. He keeps falling over. He cannot walk alone anymore.'

I nodded. It was the next stage for them.

'Who wants to play the drum?' asked Nicola holding up a small djembe. A new resident reached out, and started to hit the drum softly. Some people beside her started to clap as Nicola strummed 'Island in the Sun'. Lily nodded her head in time to the rhythm. At the end of the song Nicola asked, 'What song does Lily want to sing?' I knew what would make this day perfect for her. 'You Are My Sunshine,' I called out across the room.

Lily sang the whole song with her eyes closed. She stretched out her arms, lifted her head and sang, 'You'll never know, dear, how much I love you.' Tears trickled down her cheeks, 'Oh please don't take my sunshine away.' When she had finished singing everyone clapped and Lily opened her eyes and blinked. She had been an actor in her youth and I think, for a moment, she thought she was back on stage. She said, 'Thank you, thank you,' and bowed her head. She looked at everyone, flicked her hair back, laughed and said thank you again.

'One more song,' announced Nicola. It was almost time for lunch. Pat's voice shot across the room before anyone else could say a word. 'The Anniversary Song.'[23]

As the mysterious, sacred sound of the flute filled the room I heard Pat's voice; so sweet, so clear, so full of grief and love and courage and sorrow. 'Oh, how we danced, on the night we were wed, we vowed our true love though a word wasn't said.' Sam struggled to stand and Pat helped him. They began to dance as Pat continued to sing. '. . . Could we but recall that sweet moment sublime, We'd find that our love is unaltered by time.'

48
·

FINDING THE MOTHER
I ALWAYS WANTED

It was 10.30 am when the elevator doors slid open and I walked directly into the Residential Care Unit. About twenty residents sat in the lounge area sipping tea and nibbling on cinnamon apple cake. I could smell the warmed cake as I walked in, and I scanned the sedate, wrinkled faces for Lily, wondering whether she had wandered off again, as she was apt to do. I saw her sitting in front of the television. She was perched atop a small brown coffee table, one leg crossed over the other like a model in a photo shoot. I began to walk towards her and then stopped myself. *Just let me look at this scene.* She was oblivious to everyone in the room, engrossed in her tea and the television, but had placed herself right in the middle of the room. Her back was towards me and all I saw was her leather jacket and the strap of her ever-present brown handbag slung over one shoulder. Things had not changed that much. I walked over to her.

She turned to me and her face lit up with a huge smile. The first thing I noticed were her eyebrows: the most vibrant, stunning, pink eyebrows I had ever seen.

Lily loved to pencil in her eyebrows. She had been doing it for as long as I could remember. Soft, feathery brown strokes that framed the eyes and accentuated her whole face. Putting on her own makeup was still something she liked to do but she had stopped looking in a mirror. Whenever she had the urge, she would rummage through her well-stocked handbag for a pen, a coloured felt pen or a lipstick. All these transformed in Lily's hands to become an Estée Lauder eyebrow pencil.

She must have found a pink felt pen and decided it was the right thing to use. Her eyebrows were perfectly shaped. I tried my best not to raise my own eyebrows at the sight of her. She raised her arms with her usual heartfelt appreciation and thanked God that I had arrived.

Walking to her room became a march as she sang the words of a World War I song, 'I had a good job for fifty bob and I left, left, left right left . . .'

As we entered her room I casually mentioned that her eyebrows were an interesting colour today. She looked in the mirror.

'Jesus Christ!' she screamed. That was all it took. We began to laugh uncontrollably. When Lily laughed, she did it with every fibre of her being. Her shoulders laughed, her belly laughed, her face opened up like a six-month-old child and the tears would start trickling down her cheeks. We spent the next ten minutes oscillating between Lily peeking at herself in the mirror and then exploding into new fits of laughter. The inevitable rush to the toilet was the only thing that dragged her away from the mirror.

Slowly, using some makeup remover, we transferred the pink ink from Lily's eyebrows to the tissue. I massaged her face with moisturiser, gently, tenderly. She closed her eyes and disappeared into the moment. She looked like a child. Innocent, open, vulnerable.

This was a new experience. Though one of my past careers had been as a beautician, Lily had never let me touch her face. I had offered to give her a facial when I opened a small clinic, but she never came. And now here I was, not only touching her face, not only massaging her as I had wanted to do almost thirty years ago, but being received—totally, completely, wholly received.

49
.

I'M MARRIED?

Lily was doing well by now and I wanted to take her out. I wondered how she would cope if we returned to the shopping centre where she used to live. Would she remember any of the shops? Would she become confused if long-ago friends approached, expecting her to know them? Would she cope with the traffic and busy pedestrian footpaths? Would I unravel the good work we had done to give Lily a calm and peaceful place to live in, by taking her so close to her former home?

She was delighted to be going out. I carefully put on her makeup and took out of her handbag just enough tissues so that it could close. She climbed into the car and, surprisingly, she remembered how to buckle up her seatbelt. Things were going well.

We found a parking spot without any trouble. Another good sign. Lily had walked these streets for over forty years and I wondered whether she would start to connect to something. We looked into dress shops, the greengrocer and then the chemist. Everything was new and exciting. Lily was having a ball. Many people recognised her and seemed overjoyed to see Lily after so long. They commented on how great she looked and she slipped into her natural talent of keeping up appearances.

She responded to everyone as if she knew them.

'You look great.' *You look great too.*

'How have you been?' *You must come and have dinner with us soon.*

'Oh, how are you?' *Look how good your skin looks. Whatever you're doing, don't stop.*

After 'old friends' walked away she turned to me and in a loud voice said, 'I don't know who the hell that was,' to which we both rolled our eyes and laughed conspiratorially. As we stood at the traffic lights Lily turned around and noticed an attractive, white-haired, middle-aged man, waiting to cross the road.

'He looks nice for you. Do you want him?'

'Mummy!!! Shhh. No, I don't want him. I'm married and you're married too.'

'I'm married? What are you talking about?'

'Of course you're married.'

'Who married me?'

'Mummy, you are married to Lionel.'

'Oh, I forgot about Lionel.'

We exploded into gales of unrestrained laughter. We both held onto the traffic light and whooped and screamed together. We missed the green light, which made us collapse ever further into abandoned mirth. I could not have dreamed a more wonderful time with my mother.

50
·

WANDERING DOESN'T MEAN YOU'RE LOST

Wandering is normal behaviour for people with dementia. The act of wandering in a dementia unit includes wandering up and down hallways, wandering in and out of each other's rooms, wandering into the kitchen, the storeroom, staff meetings, and wandering in and out of each other's bedrooms, sometimes collecting things along the way.

People with dementia may think they are somewhere and forget where they were going. It may be that they are bored, or simply used to going for long walks. It may be they are searching for someone or something from their past: a friend and partner, a child. Some people may think they need to go to work or, depending on the type of dementia, they may have a hallucination or dream something and think it is real.

Wandering, along with gathering or hoarding, is typical behaviour. The boundary between what is thought and what is acted upon becomes more and more blurred as dementia progresses. We may see something that looks interesting, want it but know that we cannot take it, whereas someone with dementia will see something that is interesting and naturally reach out for it. That became embarrassingly obvious when Lily went shopping and saw a lipstick she liked or a bar of soap or a block of chocolate. These and more would find their way into her handbag. It was a miracle that she was never arrested for shoplifting.

I saw Lily leaving one of the resident's rooms, hunched over and appearing to carry a great load. She almost walked past me but stopped when she heard my voice. 'What's in your bag, Mama?'

She squeezed her bag closer to her chest and mumbled, 'Nothing.'

I walked beside her and asked, 'Can I have a look?'

We sat at the table and I waited. She looked around and nodded at a resident. I realised she had forgotten she was going to show me what was inside her handbag.

I repeated, 'What's in your bag, Mama?'

'Nothing.'

'Can I have a look?'

She pulled at the zipper and it opened. The compressed contents seemed to spring to life and sigh in relief, like a woman releasing herself from her corset at the end of the day.

She pulled out a TV remote control and put it onto the table. All in all, fourteen television remote controls appeared out of her bag. I made a joke that she really must love watching TV. She didn't laugh. 'Shall we go and put them all back, Mama?' I asked.

'No.' And with that she began to gather them up quickly, stuffing them all back in her handbag. I realised that no one in the whole Residential Care Unit would be able to watch television that day. One of the nurses was watching and started to laugh. I couldn't help myself. I began to laugh and then Lily joined in. The situation became uproariously funny.

Lily has always loved her handbags. As dementia progressed, still living at home, she would hide her various Gucci, Versace and Louis Vuitton bags in obscure places. We spent hours and hours looking for them. When she moved into the Residential Care Unit, we felt it would be less confusing if she had only one handbag. Inside this handbag—when it was not exploding with television remote controls—she carried tissues and serviettes, pieces of paper and lipsticks, five or six combs, and old business cards. She began to carry around a bra, a silk nightie and, most surprisingly, Claire's breast prosthesis. She refused to give the prosthesis back. Claire, however, seemed not to be too concerned about the situation.

Lily's bag held her world together in a manageable container.

51

CELEBRATING WHAT IS NOT LOST

So much emphasis is placed on what is lost
through dementia that it is easy to forget how
to celebrate the person who still lives on.

Lily continued to smile at everyone who smiled at her. She won the hearts of all the kitchen staff at the Residential Care Unit by telling them how wonderful they were. She never lost the ability to charm people with her compliments and friendliness and as she looked into the eyes of whoever she spoke to, there was no mistaking her sincerity. She also never lost her feistiness, impatience and sense of humour.

Barbecues

The barbecue had been heating up all morning. Some residents were already outside walking in the garden and some were sitting on the wooden benches, drinking in the first day of spring. Everyone was pale after the long winter and their old wrinkled skin seemed to unfurl and soften under the warming rays.

Lily had been uninterested in food for months. She had lost so much weight I could feel her bony skeleton under her clothes. 'Not much of you left, Mama,' I said, and she agreed. She knew she had become painfully thin but over the year she had lost her sense of smell and with it her appetite.

For some reason, though, the smell of meat cooking on the barbecue caught Lily's attention. I wondered whether some smells had been lost and others had in fact remained. I had forgotten that Lily loved a good barbecue. When her plate arrived she picked up her fork and knife and began to devour her sausage and steak with surprising gusto.

She had not lost her impeccable table manners. When I was a child, meals together with Lily and Lionel were rare. Donna and I ate in the kitchen hours before Lionel arrived home from work, and if they were not eating out for dinner, Lily and Lionel would eat dinner together in the dining room after we had gone to bed. Our bedroom was next to the dining room and we would hear their muffled chatting through the wall. Birthdays were different. On special days we were allowed to eat at the 'big table' in the dining room and we were expected to dress nicely for the occasion.

'Put your fork and knife down while you are chewing.'

'Take your elbows off the table.'

'Don't talk with your mouth full.'

'Don't slurp, burp or laugh too much.'

(Lily always put a stop to me laughing too much. She sincerely believed that if I laughed too much, I would get an asthma attack.)

Although there was a sense of excitement around eating together, the effort to eat 'as if you are dining with the Queen', dampened my enthusiasm considerably. All those rules seemed to pour out and over the perfectly set table and mire us in repressive etiquette.

Lily put her knife and fork down and began to talk.

'I like the . . . the . . . ,' she struggled to find the word.

'Steak?' I suggested.

'Yes, the steak.'

I added, 'Isn't this delicious?' and Lily agreed.

'Absolutely delicious.' She looked around, 'What a wonderful day. I'll never forget this day. Never!'

I was leaning on the table when Lily reached across and took hold of my elbow. For a moment I thought she was going to push it off. Instead she stroked my arm and told me that she loved me.

'I love you too, Mama.'

She picked up her fork and stabbed a piece of sausage, sloshed some tomato ketchup all over it, and ate it voraciously. Lily had found her appetite. Perhaps she had never really lost it. Perhaps it was simply waiting for a barbecue.

Rushing

People who know me will tell you I refuse to rush or be rushed. As punctual as I am, I would rather be late than rush. I know where this inflexibility comes from. It is in rebellious response to having a mother who was always rushing.

As my five-year-old feet skimmed the road, Lily held my tiny hand and dragged me across the road, against the red light, dodging oncoming traffic. She yelled at the top of her voice, 'Do what I say, don't do what I do,' as soon as we got to the other side of the road. I never knew if we were going to make it to the other side and sometimes would even close my eyes and just run. To this day, I don't like crossing busy roads. She may have been running late for an appointment, or coffee with a friend; it mattered not. Lily was always in a hurry to get somewhere.

We knew Lily was settling down when she began to rush around the Residential Care Unit. Of course there was nowhere to go, but she was going regardless. She had no patience to sit for any length of time and quickly became irritated if someone lingered around her. She would jump up, say, 'Goodbye, good luck and carry on,' and briskly walk away.

One day she was in such a hurry to get somewhere, she flew right past me. I called out, 'Mummy, where are you going?'

She called back, 'I'll be going when I come back.'

Oh, well, see you then . . .

Taking charge

Lily and Lionel walked hand in hand every day of their lives. No matter where they went, they held hands. Of course, when Lily moved into the Residential Care Unit Lionel was not there and so Lily made friends with Clara and they walked everywhere holding hands. After a creative morning of painting on tiles, Lily and Clara walked back into the Residential Care Unit. Some of the residents had chosen not to do the activity and others were not capable of doing something like that and so they were sitting quietly on chairs in front of the television. Lily stood in the middle of the room and looked at everyone staring ahead or sleeping. In utter disgust she strode over to the Clinical Director and shouted, 'Everyone is crazy here!'

Turning around, she grabbed Clara's hand. 'Come on, Lionel, let's get out of here.' Together they marched down the hall.

52
·

I COULD HAVE DANCED ALL NIGHT

As a high court judge he must have been impressive. A wild mop of white hair and dazzling blue eyes that positively shone with insight. He had been a resident of the Residential Care Unit long before Lily had arrived. No words had passed his lips in over six months. Alzheimer's had now taken all words away. He was sitting in a large armchair when I arrived and one of the nurses was gently coaxing him to stand up. Standing had become so challenging that Adrian could no longer do it without assistance. I walked past him, heading towards the music room where Lily and Lionel were waiting for the diversional dance therapist, Maria, to arrive.

I sat down next to them and Adrian arrived slowly, being led by a nurse who directed him to sit down next to me. Maria put on Dean Martin and we started tapping our feet to 'Mambo Italiano'.

Then Doris Day started singing, 'By the light . . . of the silvery moon, I want to spoon, To my honey I'll croon love's tune . . .'. Lionel stood up and Lily slipped into his arms. They moved around the room, gliding effortlessly as only those who have been dancing together for fifty-five years are able to do. As

I watched them move, I felt something brush against my arm. Adrian had stood up, without any assistance, and was reaching out his hand. I took it and we too began to dance. He was smiling and swaying from one foot to another. I ducked under his arm and, holding one hand, came up underneath to face him. He burst into a smile. I sang the words as I danced with him. I sang to him.

. . . Honey moon,
Keep a-shining in June,
Your silv'ry beams will bring love's dreams,
We'll be cuddlin' soon,
By the silvery moon.[24]

I looked around and realised everyone was dancing. Tears were rolling down Adrian's cheeks, trickling around his upturned mouth and landing plop, onto the front of his shirt. His eyes were shining with joy. The music ended and I motioned Adrian back to his chair, but he would not sit down. 'What is it, Adrian? Is there something you want?'

With the greatest effort he lifted his now weary, lead-weight arm and placed it on my shoulder. I stepped a little closer, not knowing what Adrian was doing. He leant forward and kissed my cheek.

'Thank you, Adrian. I loved dancing with you.' He whispered something. I know he did. I heard it. I just couldn't catch the word, but I caught the meaning and for a few moments we stood very still and just looked into each other's eyes.

53
BROKEN HIPS AND MENDED HEARTS

I could have set my clock to it: 7 am without fail the phone would ring. It mattered not that I had spent the past five hours soothing one child with asthma and had been feeding newborn twins half the night. It was irrelevant that it might be Sunday morning when we were sleeping in and that I had repeatedly requested she not ring so early. So, for a brief moment, as the phone was ringing, I thought it was Lily.

'Hello?'

'Hello, this is Beverley, from the Residential Care Unit where your mother lives.'

'Yes?'

'She has had a fall.'

'Is she okay?'

'I am ringing to tell you that she is on her way to the hospital.'

'Oh my God, what happened?'

'Well, um, er . . . actually we don't know. We just found her lying in the hall. She must have fallen. Maybe she was feeling dizzy. She was in a lot of pain so we think she may have broken her hip.'

'Dizzy? She's never been dizzy in her life!'

'I'm sorry but it was an unobserved incident.'

I wanted to scream, *How in God's name can you not know what happened? You were meant to protect my mother. This shouldn't have happened.*

'Is anyone with her now? What hospital?'

'The ambulance has picked her up and she will be at Prince of Wales hospital in about five minutes.'

I slowly put the phone down. As I hung up I realised I had not said goodbye. Carefully, with enormous effort, I called my sister. Her gentle, calm voice soothed me. 'I'll meet you at the hospital,' she said.

Hospital emergency rooms are large, cold and sterile places. Rows of broken people with dazed expressions lie on metal beds covered in white sheets that have been branded with the hospital logo. Wires and tubes hang off bleeping machines, and sharp needles are inserted into soft flesh. Grey-blue curtains suspended from steel semi-circular rods give the illusion of privacy. But there is no privacy in hospital. Charts with every detail of your life hang exposed at the end of each bed, and every interaction and decision, every rise and fall of fluid intake and output, and every heartbeat is meticulously documented from the moment you become 'the patient'.

I saw Lily the minute I walked through the heavy double doors. She looked like she had just done four rounds with Muhammad Ali. Her right eye was smeared with violent streaks of turquoise and purple. Someone appeared to have gone berserk with the latest eyeshadows. The colour rose up and over her right eyebrow where it deepened into a dark, indigo-violet that lifted off her face into a golfball-sized swelling.

She smiled.

'Mama! Did you fall?'

'Yes, I think so,' she mumbled, and then tried to get out of bed. Lionel was sitting next to her. As her bed was so high he could only see a few inches above the mattress as he stretched his arm across the cotton blanket to reach Lily's hand.

His lined face was a sickly pale grey, and his red-rimmed eyes revealed his concern. Lily tried to move closer to him but she fell back as a lightning bolt of pain shot through her body. She screamed out and my blood suddenly fell to sub-zero and stung my veins.

'Mama, you had a fall and have a broken leg.' I wasn't sure she knew where her hip was anymore; saying 'leg' was easier for her to understand.

'I have a broken leg,' she repeated and closed her eyes.

Donna began to sing. Her voice floated up and around Lily's bed. She sang a song of hope and joy that Lily loved. I joined in and so did Lionel.

'*Oseh shalom bimromav hu ya'aseh shalom aleinu v'al kol Yisrael-v'imru Amen.*'[25] (May there be abundant peace from heaven, and life, for us and for all the world.)

Our voices formed a sacred caul that wrapped and protected us from the mundane chaos of the Emergency Room. We did not notice a young, dark-haired doctor pull back the curtain until he had been standing watching us in silence for a few moments. Seeing us singing together, he appeared to be deeply moved. I even thought I saw his eyes glisten a little, but I couldn't be sure. When we finished singing he introduced himself as the orthopaedic registrar in charge of Lily. Perhaps he was not as young as I first imagined. They say you really know *you're* getting old when doctors look like they should still be in school uniform.

'Lily,' he began in a light yet knowledgeable voice, 'you have a fracture of the right hip and we will need to operate.' He began to explain what they were going to do, where they were going to take her and how long her recovery might take, but of course

Lily had no idea what he was talking about. In her inimitable way, however, she gave the impression she was following every word and nodded at exactly the right moments. It was only when he asked her how old she was that she looked around for Lionel to help her. The doctor continued to ask more questions. 'So, Lily, what actually happened? Where does it hurt? Can you wiggle your toes?'

None of these questions was of any use because Lily simply could not understand them. Eventually, unable to remain silent for another second, I said, 'Doctor, you know, Lily has Alzheimer's disease and she really doesn't understand what you are saying to her. If you tell her you are going to make her better, or that she will be all right, she will accept that.'

'Yes, I know all that but we have to tell the patient exactly what is happening.'

He turned back to Lily and repeated his question, 'Where does it hurt?'

She was becoming agitated, confused and even more incoherent than usual.

'Please, Doctor,' I begged, 'she doesn't know how to answer you.'

He must have realised his questions were pointless because he excused himself, saying he would be back soon.

Donna and I just looked at each other. It was one thing for an elderly person to have fallen and broken their hip; it was another thing completely to have broken a hip and to also have dementia. We both knew Lily had suddenly become part of a system that simply did not understand this. She was going to need us to protect her now, more than ever.

It was only eight o'clock according to the large clock hanging above the nurses' station. I rummaged through my handbag to find my mobile phone. I wanted to talk to my boys. The phone rang for a long time and I was about to hang up when a sleepy voice on the other end mumbled, 'Hello?'

It was then I realised it was Sunday morning and I had just woken my own teenage son. Sometimes you just have to call your child, no matter what time it is.

54

·

YOU SILLY BILLY

What the heck? My car had already exceeded the free two-hour parking limit, so why not just do my shopping before driving home? Parking near the hospital was impossible, unless you arrived before nine o'clock. The underground supermarket parking station was as close as I could find.

Walking down the aisles was strangely soothing. I had been sitting by Lily's hospital bed all day and was glad to be out of the drab, four-bed room with its creamy curls of weathered paint peeling off the walls. I had spent the day trying to explain in one-syllable words to Lily why she was in pain, why people were sticking needles into her arm, and why she was not allowed to get out of bed.

Darling, you fell over.

She was shocked and upset and repeated, 'I fell over?' every time I told her.

Eventually, exhausted by the repetition, I realised I was doing nothing to help Lily by telling her what happened over and over again. I changed the tone of my voice and added, 'You silly billy,' to the end of the sentence.

Darling, you fell over, you silly billy. She laughed and closed her eyes. For a while she could now let herself rest.

The doctors told us the operation had gone well. Having dementia and a broken hip, however, means that nothing, absolutely nothing, goes easily. She woke up in fear, panic and utter confusion. I was told, as they wheeled her back into her room after the surgery, that she had to be given medication to calm down. By the time I saw her she was groggy and floating in some drug-induced world.

Every time a nurse came around, I armoured myself for Lily's terrified reaction. Even having her blood pressure taken caused her to scream in fear and flail around to protect herself from these tormentors in their blue-and-white uniforms. I tried to explain to the nurses that the more words they used, the more agitated Lily would become. They told me, 'We know what to do.'

In the middle of one such long, complicated and high-volume explanation about the need to change Lily's dressings (dementia does not mean they are deaf!) my mother showed the nurse exactly what she thought of her approach and screamed, 'I'm getting out of here,' and proceeded to pull out her drains, drips, and catheter and anything else that tied her to the bed. In a calm voice that was intended to sound peaceful but came across as flat and dull, I held her hands and tried to talk to her.

'Mama, I'm here. I'm right here with you. You are in hospital. You broke your leg. It's okay. They want to help you.'

She looked at me and screamed. She spat out, 'You are horrible. Horrible. HORRRRRRRIBLE.'

I looked at her. 'I know, I am horrible.'

'You are horrible.'

'I am horrible.'

'You are horrible.'

'Horrible . . .'

'Horrible.'

'Horrible . . .'

'Horrible.'

And we kept this up, getting softer and softer, until every-thing was back in place, all the drains and tubes, and she fell asleep with me stroking her swollen brow.

55

LEAH

As I pushed my trolley down the aisle I felt the smile before I saw who it belonged to. Turning, I noticed a soft plastic doll with a pale pink velvet bonnet gathered around her face. I smiled back and then shot an awkward sideways glance in the hope that no one had seen what I had just done. I picked her up and realised I wanted to buy her for my mother.

It is strange to buy a doll for your mother. It's like turning time inside out. I had bought dolls for my children when they were ill or in hospital but buying a doll for my mother—that felt seriously strange.

I nonchalantly tossed the doll into the trolley and decided I would think about it as I completed my shopping. Would Lily have a sudden lucid moment and think I was patronising her? Would she be offended? I picked up the doll to take a closer look and gave it a squeeze. A gorgeous baby's laugh bubbled out of her soft padded body and this time two nearby shoppers turned and smiled at the doll.

'Okay,' I whispered under my breath. 'I'll buy you.'

I arrived early the next day, the doll safely hidden from view in a green shopping bag, just in case I changed my mind. Lily's bruised faced had changed; the bruise appeared to be slipping down her face and neck like a slow, muddy avalanche. Her joy at seeing me brought us both to tears.

'I brought you something, Mama.' The doll slipped out of the bag and I handed it to her with as much respect as I could muster.

She instantly dissolved into tears. She held the doll to her lips and kissed it over and over, saying, 'I love you. I love you, so much. I love you. I love you.' The nurse carrying a bedpan out from behind the curtains of the neighbouring patient poked her head around the corner to see what all the 'I love you's' were about. At that moment Lily squeezed the doll and it began to laugh. Lily's eyes opened so wide I thought she was going to faint. But no, she too began to laugh. It was the kind of laugh that no matter how much your body hurts it doesn't matter because it's too delicious to stop. She squeezed again. Tears rolled down her cheeks.

'What's her name, Mama?' She tried to say a name. 'L . . . Li . . . L . . .'

I said the first name that came into my head. Leah. 'Is it Leah?'

'Yes,' she said. 'Leah.' And then came a moment of lucidity. 'Leah was my mother's name,' she said.

'Yes, Mummy, Leah was your mother's name.'

And for the second time in two days, I stroked her swollen brow and she fell asleep. This time holding Leah to her heart.

56
·

YOU JUST DON'T GET IT, DO YOU?

Donna and I spent the next few days alternately sitting beside Lily from early morning till late afternoon. Sometimes we would pass each other in the hall as one was leaving and the other arriving and we would either smile or sigh, depending on what kind of day it had been. The nursing staff continued to explain to Lily every detail of what they intended to do and how long it would take and what she should expect, and no matter how many times I explained to them that she didn't understand, they insisted it was protocol.

On the day Lily's catheter was removed she was told she would have to use the pan or they would put the catheter back in. Such verbal threats were so commonplace in hospital that I doubt whether the nurses ever realised how punitive and intimi-dating they sounded. Later that day Lily announced she wanted to 'do wee wee'.

I told a nurse, and suddenly it was, 'All hands, man your battle stations.'

Two nurses arrived, sleeves rolled up, and Lily was lifted from her bed onto a commode chair. Pain gripped her hip and she screamed loudly. Lying in the bed opposite was Margaret, a partially deaf church cleric, who had tripped whilst leaving church three weeks ago and broken her leg. She rolled her eyes. I had overheard her telling her equally deaf visitor that morning, 'That lady acts like a spoilt brat.'

Lily's gown flared open behind her, revealing her bare bottom. The nurse marched the commode chair down the hall and I ran after, trying to pull Lily's gown around her tiny, exposed body. Lily held onto the cold metal arm rails of the chair, unaware of what was happening or even where she was going.

'I'll stay with her,' I offered.

'She'll be right, deary. We'll bring her back when she's done,' replied the nurse without looking in my direction. The bathroom door slowly closed and I returned to Lily's room to wait. The minutes ticked away. Two minutes, three, four, five minutes. *What's going on?*

'Just go to the toilet, Lily! Just do it. Come on. Just go to the toilet. Be a good girl and hurry up!' I heard the impatient, irritated voice as I approached the bathroom.

'What's happening?' I asked.

'She just won't do it. I'll have to call the doctor and get her catheterised again,' she threatened. 'Come on, dear. Just go to the toilet.'

I looked at Lily, who was trying to get off the commode. She was trying to 'go' somewhere. She was putting all her energy into 'going' but she couldn't and was confused and upset, not to mention in obvious pain.

I lost it.

'Do you nurses have any training at all in working with people with dementia?'

'Yes, we do,' snapped the nurse.

'Well, it's clearly not enough. For God's sake, she doesn't understand what you want her to do. Can't you see she is trying to "go" to a toilet? She doesn't realise she is sitting over it.'

I squeezed myself into the bathroom past the nurse and went over to Lily.

'Mummy, Mummy, look at me. Darling, this chair has a hole in it.' I showed her. 'So you can do a wee now. It will go down into the toilet.'

She couldn't connect the feeling to the action. Nothing happened. Suddenly I remembered something Lily did when I was a child. I put on the tap and as the water tricked down the sink I made a pshhh pshhh sound. 'Pshhhhh . . . Pshhh . . . Pshhhhh . . .'

'I'll come back later,' said the nurse as she spun around and strode out of the bathroom.

'Pshhhhhh . . . Pshhhh . . .'

I made up a song about doing a wee and danced around the bathroom singing.

'I've got to do a wee, I've got to do a wee, Hey ho the dairy-o, I've got to do a wee.'

Nothing.

'Let's have a warm shower, Mama.'

Donna arrived at that moment. We turned on the shower tap and warm water streamed down. We kicked off our shoes and pushed her commode chair into the water. 'Don't wet my hair,' admonished Lily. She hated having wet hair. As the warm water caressed her skin, we made 'mmmm' and 'ahhh' sounds together. I suggested we both splash the next nurse to walk into the bathroom. Lily eagerly agreed. We were now conspirators and I secretly glanced over at the door . . . hoping.

'Oh, how wonderful.' Lily closed her eyes and gently her body remembered what to do.

With Lily dried and dressed in a fresh gown, we wheeled her back to bed. Donna and I smiled and hugged for a long time. It was one of those days. I started to leave when I saw Donna place her hands on each side of Lily's brow and stroke her with feathery softness.

'*Ay lalula, sheina kindela, Ay lalula, sheina kindela, Ay lalula lula lula lu, Ay lalula sheina kindela.*' Her sweet voice soothing Lily with the Yiddish lullaby she had sung to us when we were children. I imagine my grandmother had sung it to Lily when she was a child too. And now, the daughter sings the mother her own lullaby. *Go to sleep, go to sleep my darling child. Go to sleep, Go to sleep, Go to sleep.*

Lily shut her eyes and drifted off to sleep. Donna looked up and we saw each other remembering, remembering a long time ago.

57
·

RESPECT

The famous psychotherapist Sigmund Freud said the aim of wit
is the pleasurable or hostile satisfaction obtained in telling jokes.[26]
Freud added that joking is essentially a social activity requiring
the presence of a second party.

> **It is easier to laugh at ourselves in the presence
> of others than when we are alone.**

Through play with words and thoughts, jokes enable adults
to rediscover the infantile part of themselves that allows them
to be silly, immature and playful. Jokes help us make light of
our pain and troubles. We are able to make fun of ourselves and
minimise that which we most fear.

Lily was sitting with her back to me as I entered the Residential
Care Unit. Since the fall, she had been confined to a wheelchair.
Occasionally the staff would take her up and down the corridor
with her walker.

When I reached her, she stretched out her arms, fell into my chest and started to cry. She was happy to see me, but also distressed. Her tears needed acknowledgment.

'Are you sad today, Mama?'

'Yes.'

'Did something happen?'

And then a jumble of words poured out; phrases that held the key . . . but which word was the key? She pointed to the nurses' station and then tried to explain, 'This one . . . she didn't say . . . do . . . and it wasn't right, not right . . . all this,' she motioned around the whole room.

'Let's go for a walk, Mama.'

It was always good to get out of the Residential Care Unit, if for no other reason but to see the delight on Lily's face as I pressed the code, 5, 4, 3, 2, OK and the door magically opened.

We walked out of the Residential Care Unit, past the coffee shop and dining hall, and wandered into a light, airy lounge room with pale green couches facing the large floor-to-ceiling windows. In the far left of the room sat a small piano. A group of residents who lived in the independent section of the home had gathered there, to enjoy an hour of joke-telling.

Lily and I wandered into the room and I asked her whether she would like to sit down and listen for a moment. The lady reading the jokes stopped and looked at us.

'Do you want to walk through?' she asked with some irritation.

'No, we want to sit down, if that is all right?'

'Oh,' she shrugged, 'very well.'

Lily walked unsteadily, leaning heavily on her walker. I thought I saw some people whisper to their neighbours, but I probably imagined it. Some of the people had known Lily long ago when she was young, vibrant, beautiful and busy with her social life. No one said hullo.

Lily sat down and smiled her glorious smile at me. We cuddled close. Everyone was laughing at the jokes. Some were very funny and others not so, but Lily laughed and hugged me at the end of every joke. It didn't matter whether she understood the words, the atmosphere was lighthearted and her mood had turned.

The next joke was more a piece of 'funny' advice. I listened, waiting for the end so that Lily and I would laugh again together.

'How to stay young . . .

'One—throw out nonessential numbers. This includes age, weight and height. Let the doctor worry about them. That is why you pay him/her. Two—keep only cheerful friends. The grouches pull you down. Three—keep learning. Learn more about the computer, crafts, gardening, whatever. Never let the brain be idle. An idle mind is the devil's workshop. And the devil's name is Alzheimer's.'

I was stunned. I could not move or breathe. Did I really hear a joke calling Alzheimer's the devil's name? A woman on my right made a sharp intake of breath. I slowly turned to look at Lily. There she was, sweet and innocent, smiling away and squeezing my hand. *Of course*, I reminded myself, *she didn't understand the words*.

'This is wonderful. You are wonderful. I love you,' she beamed at me. I smiled and hugged her back. The woman with the microphone finished and left. It was time to go. Lily stood up and held onto her walker. She stood so straight that I felt I, too, needed to stand tall beside her. I turned to those assembled and said goodbye.

No one responded. Eyes diverted in a vain attempt to pretend they had not noticed us.

I know they were frightened by what they saw: Lily, painfully shuffling past acquaintances she no longer recognised. I know that in some strange way their fear convinced them that if someone like Lily was out of sight, the dreaded devil whose name was Alzheimer's would never tap them on the shoulder.

I felt a great surge of protective love come over me. Later, I wrote a complaint to the social worker in charge. I stood high on my soapbox and said that compassion is not a weakness and Alzheimer's is not contagious. In her professional way she acknowledged me and said she would find out how the joke had come to be told. Nothing ever came of that. I let it be.

But it was not the joke. It was the fear that permeated that room the moment we walked in, and caused everyone present to avert their eyes. If I could say one thing to the people in that room it would be, *It's okay. I understand. My mother also averted her eyes to things she wanted to avoid.* I would also add something else. In the fourth century BCE, Plato wrote, 'May I do to others as I would that they should do unto me.' I imagine if we did that, we would probably laugh a great deal more, even without an hour of jokes.

58
·

WHEN VALIDATION
GOES OUT THE WINDOW

'You *have* to eat your sandwich or you *won't* get ice cream,' the loud, threatening voice rang out through the Residential Care Unit. I looked around and saw a tall, thin, curly-haired nurse admonishing Patty, a Holocaust survivor, who had become a school principal and author of a number of best-selling non-fiction books. Patty repeated, 'No, no, no . . .' and turned her head away.

The nurse turned to Lily and repeated the sentence. Lily instantly became angry; she pushed her plate away and tried to get up from the table.

'I don't . . . don't you speak . . . I'm getting out of here . . .' Although the words came out jumbled, her intention was perfectly clear. The nurse pushed the plate back in front of Lily. I felt suddenly paralysed.

I'm coming, I screamed in silence and took a super-human stride forward.

What I considered saying in that instant between then and now was, *How dare you speak to these adults as if they were recalcitrant children?* But what came out was, 'Excuse me, excuuuuuse me, WHY ARE YOU YELLING?'

She jumped.

A word of advice to the livid, fuming and irate: if you want to ask someone why they are yelling, it is advisable to ask the question in a relatively quiet manner or else the point is lost.

She began to turn pink from the chest up. I watched the colour rise and become a patchwork of blotches over her neck. 'What?' She looked genuinely shocked.

'They don't have to finish their lunch,' I said in a seething whisper. 'They are adults. Grown-up people. You are speaking to them as if they are naughty children.'

'But—but—they have to eat,' she stuttered. Lily had pushed her chair away from the table, saying, 'Goodbye, good luck and carry on.' Patty stood up and also left the table.

As a tray carrying six bowls of vanilla ice cream was being served to the neighbouring table, I heard Patty say to no one in particular, 'I hate ice cream.'

> **Adults with dementia in nursing homes who are talked to like children are more resistant to care.**

'The style of communication that we use with people with Alzheimer's influences how they feel about themselves and how well they respond to those providing care,' says Dr Sam Fazio of the US Alzheimer's Association.[27]

Addressing the growing prevalence of Alzheimer's in the world today, he stresses that it is 'increasingly important for healthcare providers, caregivers and families to understand the effect Alzheimer's has on communication . . . more importantly, the impact their communication may have on the individual's quality of life.'

The growing population of adults with Alzheimer's presents complex challenges to care providers. Kristine Williams RN PhD and colleagues at the University of Kansas School of Nursing explored the relationship between how nursing home staff communicate with those with dementia and subsequent behaviours that disrupt care, or what researchers call 'resistiveness to care'. Specifically, the study examined whether nursing staff 'elder-speak' affected 'resistiveness to care' behaviours.

'Elder-speak' can be speaking more loudly than necessary, being overly caring, and controlling and infantilising communication, similar to 'baby talk'.

For example, Mrs Green enjoys the flower-arranging activity. She takes great pride in her finished arrangement. The choice of nursing staff in saying, 'Well, you are soooo clever, aren't you, Mrs Green?' or 'Well done, Mrs Green. Your arrangement is beautiful,' can have the effect of Mrs Green feeling patronised and becoming agitated or her feeling acknowledged and satisfied. Common features of elder-speak are simplified grammar and vocabulary, use of plural pronouns such as 'we' instead of 'you', and overly intimate endearments.

Resistiveness to care increases the stress of nursing staff, the length of time needed to provide care, and the costs of care. At the same time, it may actually indicate unmet needs that the person with Alzheimer's is unable to communicate in a conventional way.

Kristine Williams's study suggests that there is an association between the communication style of nursing staff and the behaviours of their patients. 'This may significantly impact nursing care and how nursing home staff should best be trained to communicate with residents with Alzheimer's,' Williams and her colleagues suggest.[28]

I remember a time Lily and I went into a clothing shop, long before she became a resident of the Residential Care Unit. She was taking clothes off the shelves and mumbling to herself. The shop assistant came over and asked whether she required any help. Lily said no. She then opened her handbag and began to stuff a t-shirt into it. 'You can't take that,' I whispered loudly. She ignored me and I said it again: 'Mum, put the t-shirt on the shelf.' She became furious and yelled at me and marched out of the shop. I ran after her but she walked away so fast it took some time to catch up. She was angry and very upset and wanted nothing to do with me.

Had I known then what I know now, I would have done it differently. I might have told her the t-shirt was the wrong colour for her. I might have offered to pay for it for her. I might have suggested she try it on first. I might have even made a joke and whispered, 'Are we going to steal the t-shirt?' I know she would have responded to one of those suggestions without being embarrassed or shamed. But, like most of us, I had to learn the hard way.

59

·

FLOURISHING

Everything changes, even those times when loss, pain and confusion become almost intolerable. This too shall pass.

After the initial numbing confusion and desperate helplessness of going into the Residential Care Unit, Lily felt so comfortable in the unit she seldom wanted to leave. On the rare occasions she did agree to go out for a drive or have a cup of coffee in a cafe, she often asked to 'go home' within an hour of leaving the unit. The routine, the music, the corridors, the contact and closeness with staff, all felt familiar and safe.

A large red plastic ball seemed to hover in the air as I entered the Residential Care Unit. Lily was sitting in a circle with a group of residents all laughing and enjoying the game. Seeing me, however, she jumped up and literally ran to greet me. I picked her up and in a moment of spontaneity, whirled her around and around. The irony of lifting my own mother off the ground and spinning with her in my arms was not lost on me.

Putting her gently down, I led her towards the door that led outside and into the garden. The garden, with its many inter-connecting paths, was full of herbs. I picked a sprig of rosemary and handed it to Lily.

'Smell it,' I said. She screwed up her nose and said she didn't like it. I picked some lemon thyme and asked her whether she liked that one. She did. We found a wooden bench next to a mint bush and sat in silence for a moment.

Lily turned to me and asked, 'How are the children?'

I was surprised; not only had she asked me a question, but such a relevant, mother sort of question. 'They are well, Mummy. Sheli is overseas and Orly is studying at university.'

'And the boys, how are they getting on?'

Now for most people this conversation would seem very normal, but for Lily it had been years since she had been able to articulate such thoughts. It seemed to me at that moment that she did not have advanced dementia at all. That perhaps we had made a mistake. We had been told that once she settled down there might be moments of lucidity. Such occurrences even have a name: flourishing. I remember when I heard that word, it sounded so positive and exciting. I actually looked forward to it happening. Now that it was happening, I was not so sure.

'Fine. They are at school and studying.'

She nodded and then in a voice that revealed a broken heart she said, 'I'm never going home again, am I?'

Nothing could have prepared me for this question. I realised my mother understood everything at that moment.

'No, Mummy. This is your home now.'

'I want to go home.'

Her eyes filled with tears and she repeated, 'Why can't I go home to Lionel?'

I answered honestly. 'Mummy, Lionel is no longer able to care for you because he is very old.'

'Lionel is old?'

'Yes, he is old. He is too old to look after you. Do you want to know how old he is?'

'Yes.'

'He is ninety years old.'

'Ninety years old? My God. When did that happen?'

She stopped talking and we just sat still for a few minutes.

A breeze blew her hair into her face and she stood up.

'I want to go home now,' she said and began to walk towards the door leading back into the Residential Care Unit. We walked in. Afternoon tea was being served. She looked around, smiled and said, 'I love it here. It's wonderful, isn't it?'

'Wonderful, Mummy.' I smiled and watched her settle into a comfortable chair.

60
·

ADJUSTING MY EYES
TO THE NEW LILY

Finding Lily was becoming more difficult. I had to really look. She had begun to blend into the room. She no longer stood out as she used to. As the lift doors opened and I stepped into the sitting room, I scanned the room. *Where is she?*

Suddenly, right in front of me, a little hand was waving. *Oh my God. I didn't recognise her.* Ironically, she still knew me. Her transformation in one year was like that of a newborn through to their first birthday, only in reverse.

Her hair was now white. Years ago I remember wondering what Lily would look like if she let her brown hair, streaked with a few rays of sunshine, go grey. I tried to imagine it, but I couldn't. It was impossible. So ingrained in me was her image, I could not change it until it changed itself.

Her skin had also become milky-white. Eighty years of loving the sun and relishing a tan were gone. They slipped away into this latest winter and forgot to come back in spring. Her pale skin yielded as I gently smoothed face cream over silky wrinkles. I could barely feel her skin. It had become so soft. She closed her eyes and smiled.

Because she had shrunk both in height and weight, trousers hung on her hipless figure like a massive boilersuit.

One of the most extraordinary changes, however, was that Lily had become still. She could now sit quietly and just be. I think that was why I often couldn't find her. Her whole energy had shifted. The frenetic get-up-and-go that made her struggle as well as shine and shimmer had transformed itself into relative stillness. Whether Lily actually felt calm, I don't know, but being with her, I felt her gentleness meet my own in a way it never had before. Of course, there were times when Lily's feisty nature took over, especially when one of the other residents was bothering her, but generally when I arrived she would be sitting peacefully in her own world. As soon as she saw me she would light up, raise her thin arms joyfully and thank God.

From being a mother who rarely acknowledged or approved of me she had become completely adoring of everything about me. Donna and I marvelled that she had long passed the stage of mere acceptance of who we were and was now in pure and unconditional love with us.

'You are so beautiful. Perfect,' she would say.

'I love you, I love you, I love you,' she would chant.

'I have always loved you,' she would declare.

'I will never forget you,' she would promise.

Donna and I were chatting about Lily and she commented that Lily could be saying all these things to her, looking deeply into her eyes, when a nurse or another visitor would catch her attention. Then she would seamlessly shift all her passion and love to that person and say everything again, with identical sincerity. We laughed. It was a sobering reality that, as Lily had become the mother we had always wanted, we were no longer the sole beneficiaries of her unconditional love.

She no longer remembers her friends, who stopped visiting her. She has no regrets or resentments left. She is no longer concerned with her appearance, or anyone else's, for that matter. She is completely honest about those whom she does not like and then a minute later is declaring undying love to them. She loves everyone who smiles at her. That is her yardstick.

Every time I visit Lily, I, too, have started to thank God. Every minute I spend with her is a blessing for me as it is for her. And that is perhaps her greatest gift. Lily is Love. So few of us can say that about ourselves, but I can say it about Lily.

61
·

EARTH, TECHNOLOGY
AND DEMENTIA

Why is dementia so prevalent in the twenty-first century? We know dementia is a physical disease. We know it usually affects the elderly, although early onset of Alzheimer's is also increasing.

Dementia can affect younger people; currently over 9,600 Australians under the age of 65 have younger onset dementia.[29]

We have even spoken about dementia as a stage of resolution before the individual dies. I would like to share another perspective. A personal hypothesis.

People with dementia are not grounded. Being grounded means being fully present: physically, emotionally and energetically. It means your mind is not wandering or pulling your energy elsewhere. Your heart and soul are not searching somewhere in the past or looking into the future. People with dementia are not grounded. They have lost their anchor. If a ship cannot put down its anchor it will float aimlessly upon the ocean. If a tree is not rooted into the earth it will fall over. If a balloon is not held firmly it will fly away.

What keeps us anchored in the here and now is our connection to the earth and its cycles. When we let go of the land, we become vulnerable to disease. Connection to the land grounds our energies. Being in and with nature connects us to our own inner stillness. It reminds us to stop and breathe. It helps us to reconnect to our soul. When we forget to notice the stars in a winter sky and the falling leaves of an old oak tree, or the dripping ice cream rolling down a child's arm, we lose contact with the earth. What keeps us anchored in the here and now is our connection to the earth, to nature and its cycles, night and day, summer, autumn, winter, spring. Much of humanity has moved from being at one with the land, into dominating the landscape.

With the rapid increase of fast computers, mobile phones, instant connections and instant disconnections, life has sped up. This wave of super-fast technology has impacted the electromagnetic energy field of the earth itself. People become agitated and little by little begin to detach from the present because it has become uncomfortable. We live in a society where multi-tasking is the norm. Research into multi-tasking has shown that the human brain simply isn't very good at spreading its energy between different things.[30] It can take on average around twenty minutes to get your mind focused on the task at hand. Start trying to do two things at once and that period of time will increase dramatically. What's more, once you get distracted from your work and break that focus, you basically have to start the whole process again.

Multi-tasking is an outgrowth of our computer- and media-oriented era. As computers and electronic devices have become higher powered and more sophisticated, the features they offer have grown in number and complexity. A mobile phone was initially just that, a mobile phone. But over time, it has become a camera, a video camera, a portable media player, a GPS device, a hand-held computer, and all kinds of other things. We seem to have a fixation in our culture with 'more is better'. But we're not so good at figuring out 'how much is enough?'

As a consequence of this unchecked and unbalanced development, those who need an anchor lose it. We have forgotten how to balance our lives through nature. People have forgotten how to connect to the earth. We are no longer aware of the cycles of the seasons. We have lost our healthy respect for the elements: fire, water, air and earth. We seem to believe that we can control everything, but of course we cannot. When we separate from the land we are at the mercy of the powerfully ungrounding forces of technology.

As people lose their connection to the land they get caught up in the 'shoulds' and 'musts' and 'have to's' of everyday life.

In time their connection to their dreams and aspirations also fades. Perhaps in this way, those with dementia become more vulnerable to the disease. Mentally they began to detach from the past as well. They lose that anchor also. One moment they are present and the next moment they are gone. As the disease progresses, connection to the present and the past becomes more fragile. One minute they are here in the present and in the next minute they are gone.

62

•

INDIA

Oren and I began to talk about taking a vacation. We had been to India a few times and loved the country. 'What do you think about inviting your father?' Oren asked. I phoned him right away and suddenly we were planning an overseas trip with my ninety-year-old father.

For weeks we debated how and when to tell Lily that we were going away. Eventually, the day before we left, we told her very simply, 'We are going to India tomorrow for a holiday.' As always she was excited and happy for us. 'Lionel is coming too. But we will be coming back soon.' She hesitated for a moment and then hugged him, wishing him a wonderful trip. We kissed her goodbye and as she no longer had any concept of time we simply repeated we would be back soon.

We travelled throughout Rajasthan for four weeks and for the first time in my life Lionel and I spent hours talking to one another. On the last day in Delhi I asked him how was he feeling about returning home.

'Ambivalent,' he replied.

'Why is that?' I asked.

He went on to tell me that he had hoped this trip would heal his aching heart. He had hoped he would not miss Lily so much after the trip. 'But I do. I don't know if I'll ever stop missing her.'

Four hours after landing he walked into the Residential Care Unit. Lily looked up from her armful of terry-towelling bibs and smiled. It took a moment to remember him. Lionel opened his arms. 'Hello, sweetheart.' Suddenly she was running into his arms. They hugged, kissed and hugged again. Then suddenly she pulled away. Her smile disappeared and she said, 'You went away. You went away without me.'

We knew Lily would miss Lionel; after all, she has never really stopped looking for him, but to tell him off was unexpected. Rather than defend himself, Lionel agreed. 'Yes, I went to India with Sharon and Oren,' and then he shared with her a story about his adventure.

Lily reproached Lionel every day. Every time he visited, his presence seemed to flick a switch and she admonished him again and again. 'You went away. You went away without me.' And every day he told her he had gone to India and told her another story about his trip. On the tenth day Lily greeted him with open arms, without any disapproval or accusation. The memory of being left behind had gone and, just to be safe, Lionel's stories of India also came to an end.

63

•

SORRY TO LEAVE YOU

Until our first child was born, Lily and Lionel had only spent five days apart. It took the birth of a grand-daughter for Lily to fly halfway around the world, but after three days she missed Lionel so much, she cut short her visit and returned home. They never left each other's side again until she moved into the Residential Care Unit.

Donna and I rarely travelled out of town at the same time. Donna visited Lily the whole time we were in India and I did the same when she went away. This weekend, however, Donna was away on a work assignment, Oren was overseas visiting three of our children and I was at a conference.

On my return I called Lionel, but as soon as I heard his voice, I knew he had been crying, and he struggled to tell me that Lily was very ill. She had not eaten for two days, he said, and had lost weight. 'I think she's doing this on purpose. I think . . .' The words were stuck and a small groan escaped his throat, 'I think she is getting herself ready to . . .' I told him I was on my way and that I would come to see him as soon as I had seen Lily. My twin sons jumped in the car with me and we headed to the Residential Care Unit.

There she was, standing alone. This tiny, frail woman, somewhat worse for wear, was my mother. I barely recognised her. She looked up and, as always, brought both hands to her chest and cried out, 'Thank you, God.'

Lily was also covered in vomit. One of the staff, who saw us embracing her, told me she was just about to change her clothes. The Residential Care Unit had had a flare-up of gastroenteritis, she explained to me.

'I'll do it,' I said. 'I'll change her.'

I have found, in these situations, it is best not to allow any thoughts of who Lily used to be to come into my mind, for in truth she was unrecognisable. She still wore a pale shadow of a bruise under her right eye. A raw wound, covered in a bloody bandage, appeared like a medal in the middle of her chest. Apparently a resident in a hurry to get past earlier that day had pushed her. She could not have weighed more than 35 kilos. She seemed also to have shrunk a few centimetres since she had moved into the Residential Care Unit, almost one year ago to the day.

'Mummy, look, here are the boys. They came to visit you.' Her face broke open into a rapturous smile and she lifted her arms to hug them. They in turn greeted their grandma warmly, not once flinching from the smell of the vomit that stained her shirt and pants.

The boys waited as I took her to her room and dressed her in a fresh clean shirt. Walking back to the lounge, oblivious to having been sick, she sang 'Pack Up Your Troubles'. I took out my mobile phone and played a few videos of Lily singing with me the previous week and she laughed and joined in. It was not her time to go yet.

She waved us goodbye and threw us kisses as we disappeared into the lift.

Lionel, on the other hand, tired and drawn and sad beyond words, opened a bottle of wine. I told him Lily had seemed okay when I visited. Better than she had been earlier in the day. He listened, his eyes staring at a patch of fluff on his dark blue trousers. I found it hard to believe I had only landed home three hours ago.

64
·

LOST AND FOUND

The realisation exploded like an acacia pod on a sweltering summer's day. How could I not have realised? The saying, 'You don't know what you've got until you've lost it' had just turned itself inside out. You don't know what you've lost until you've found it. The search was over.

For weeks I had tried to write an ending for this book. In the early days, I wondered whether someone would die and in some stereotypical way I would tie up all loose threads.

Someone did die, but it was not Lily or Lionel. In fact, they are both doing well. Lily is comfortable, settled, eating well and still greets us with joy whenever we arrive. I don't think she will ever deteriorate to the point of not recognising us. At 83 she has resumed her fast walking pace, albeit with a walker. Her broken hip only slowed her down momentarily. And Lionel has just celebrated his ninety-first birthday. He continues to do his medical consultations via the telephone and fiercely chooses to live alone.

I was visiting the children overseas when my mobile phone rang. Oren's voice softly told me that my Aunty Doris, Lily's older sister, had just passed away.

Doris was everything Lily was not. Where Lily was glamorous, Doris was homely. While Lily dressed to the nines for charity balls, Doris visited the sick and volunteered to cook for the aged. While Lily devoted herself to Lionel, Doris devoted herself to her religious community. While my parents travelled overseas to attend medical conferences in China and cruise around the Greek islands, Doris looked after my sister and me. It is her soulful chicken soup, carrot tzimmes and shortbread biscuits that we strive to imitate in our own kitchens. I loved Doris. And now she was gone.

I held the phone to my ear long after Oren had hung up. Lost in thought, I didn't notice Sheli come into the room and sit down beside me. I had loved Doris. She was the matriarch of our family for many years. It was hard to believe she was gone. As Sheli sat quietly I began to muse aloud. 'With Doris gone there's only my mum and dad left.'

Lily was the youngest of four children and Lionel the youngest of six. The babies of the family, and now, the only ones left. Lionel was a change-of-life baby, born to a mother almost fifty years old. His oldest brother was already married and had children of his own when Lionel was born. There were sixteen years between Lionel and the next sibling.

His mother, sick and tired of mothering, often left him to travel the world. Gripping life with both hands, he decided to become a doctor. Passing every exam with honours, he was awarded the university medal in medicine. No one in his family witnessed his achievements.

I once asked him what he wanted more than anything as a child, and he told me he wanted someone who would welcome him home every day. He found that person in Lily and she became his passion, perhaps even his obsession. There was little room for anyone else. Though he loved his children he never showed us. And like his parents before him, he never came to one graduation or prize-giving.

As a child I sat in my father's study by the side of his rosewood desk. I sat on the floor facing an overcrowded bookshelf that was straining under the weight of the Encyclopaedia Britannica. As he dictated his letters to other doctors into a dictaphone, I would thumb through the A-B, or the N-O or X-Y-Z volumes and try to memorise a fact that would impress him later. I don't remember one fact I memorised, but I remember being so happy sitting by his feet. One day he might ask me what I was reading and I would be prepared.

I longed for a father who would ask me questions. Over the years the longing faded until I forgot I had ever wanted a different father. When Lily and Lionel were a glamorous couple—the doctor and doctor's wife—it was Lily who shone, Lily who chattered, Lily who led the conversations and took over the room. My father would quietly sit on the sideline, whistling a Sinatra tune. That's just how it was.

Things have shifted now. Every Friday night he comes to dinner and with a little encouragement, talks about his life. He has a riveted audience. We ask him a hundred questions. Every Friday without fail we discover something new about my father; his life is a long, unfinished story that reveals a new chapter every week.

Sitting on the bed in my daughter's home I realised I had been looking for Lionel too. In many ways we all had. Out of the disorder and confusion, the pain and loss, we found the mother and the father we never had. Through dementia we have lost. And through dementia we have found.

NOTES

1 Access Economics, 2005 *Dementia Estimates and Projections: The Australian States and Territories*, Alzheimer's Australia, Canberra, 2005.

2 *World Alzheimer Report 2009*, eds Professor Martin Prince and Mr Jim Jackson, Alzheimer's Disease International, 21 September 2009, <www.alz.co.uk/research/worldreport/>, p. 38.

3 Alzheimer's Australia, PO Box 4019, Hawker ACT 2614, phone (02) 6254 4233.

4 Access Economics, *Dementia in the Asia Pacific Region: The Epidemic is Here*, Alzheimer's Australia, Canberra, 2006.

5 Thomas Moore, *Care of the Soul*, HarperCollins Publishers, New York, 1992; James Hillman, *Archetypal Psychology*, Spring Publications Inc., New York, 1997.

6 Dan Gottlieb, *Frontotemporal Dementia Caregiver Conference*, Philadelphia, PA, 2005.

7 Richard Hycner and Lynn Jacobs, *The Healing Relationship in Gestalt Therapy*, The Gestalt Journal Press, New York, 1995.

8 Anthony F. Jorm, Keith B.G. Dear and Nicole M. Burgess, 'Projections of future numbers of dementia cases in Australia with and without prevention', *Australian and New Zealand Journal of Psychiatry*, vol. 39, issue 11–12, pp. 959–963.

9 Robert H. Binstock, Stephen Garrard Post and Peter J. Whitehouse, *Dementia and Aging: Ethics, Values, and Policy Choices*, JHU Press, Baltimore, Maryland, 1992. Stephen G. Post is a professor in the Department of Bioethics at the Case Western Reserve University School of Medicine. President of the Institute for Research on

Unlimited Love, he has studied altruism and unselfish love for three decades at the interface of science, philosophy and world religions. Peter J. Whitehouse MD PhD is Director of Integrative Studies at Case Western Reserve University, as well as professor of neurology, psychiatry, neuroscience, psychology, nursing, organisational behaviour and biomedical ethics and history. Robert H. Binstock is Professor of Aging, Health, and Society at Case Western Reserve University. His primary appointment is in the Department of Epidemiology & Biostatistics in the School of Medicine. He holds secondary appointments as professor in the departments of Bioethics, Medicine, Political Science, Sociology and in the School of Nursing.

10 B. Bettelheim, afterword to C. Vegh, *I Didn't Say Goodbye*, trans. by R. Schwartz, E.P. Dutton, New York, 1984, p. 166.

11 Jane Verity, founder and CEO of Dementia Care Australia, quoted at <www.dementiacareaustralia.com>, accessed 30 September 2009. Jane has been developing her own approach to dementia care: the *Spark of Life* approach. She has worked with Tom Kitwood, the creator of Person Centred Care. She is also an advocate for the Eden Alternative and is the current Eden Alternative mentor for all Nordic countries. The Eden Alternative is an international, not-for-profit organisation dedicated to transforming care environments into habitats for human beings that promote quality of life for all involved. It is a powerful tool for inspiring wellbeing for elders and those who collaborate with them as care partners.

The Eden Alternative's principle-based philosophy empowers care partners to transform institutional approaches to care into the creation of a community where life is worth living. It is led by the internationally recognised founder, Dr William Thomas.

12 Jolene Brackey, *Creating Moments of Joy*, Purdue University Press, West Lafayette, Indiana, 2007.

13 Jane Verity, quoted at <www.dementiacareaustralia.com>, accessed 30 September 2009.

14 Terry Pratchett, *Mail Online Health*, 18 January 2009, <www.dailymail.co.uk/health/article-1070673/Terry-Pratchett-Im-slipping-away-bit-time--I-watch-happen.html>, accessed 31 August 2009.

15 The Multi-Institutional Research in Alzheimer's Genetic Epidemiology (MIRAGE) study has been funded by the United States National Institute of Aging (NIA) since 1990 and has

demonstrated that genetic factors play a major role in the development of Alzheimer's disease.

16 Cupples, L.A., Winberg, J., Beiser, A., Auerbach, S.H., Volicer, L., Cipolloni, P.B., Wells, J., Growdon, J.H., D'Agostino, R., Wolf, P.A., Farrer, L.A., 'Effects of smoking, alcohol and APOE genotype on Alzheimer's Disease: the MIRAGE study', *Alzheimer's Reports*, issue 3, 2000, pp. 105–113.

17 Copyright Peer International Corp. International copyright secured. All rights reserved. Used by permission.

18 Discussed in Alzheimer's Association, 'Dealing with guilt', fact sheet no. 516, <www.alzheimers.org.au/factsheet/516>, accessed 30 September 2009.

19 Jeanne Katzman, 'How families work to maintain conversational coherence during interactive dinner time talk', *Alzheimer's & Dementia*, vol. 4, issue 4, supplement, pp. T147–T148, July 2008.

20 Naomi Feil, *The Validation Breakthrough: Simple techniques for communicating with people with 'Alzheimer's-type dementia'*, Health Professions Press Inc., Maryland, USA, 2002.

21 Mem Fox and Julie Vivas, *Wilfrid Gordon McDonald Partridge*, Omnibus Books, Adelaide, 1984.

22 Feil, *The Validation Breakthrough*.

23 'The Anniversary Song' by Al Jolson and Saul Chaplin © 1946 Mood Music Division, Shapiro, Bernstein and Co. Inc., New York. Copyright renewed. International copyright secured. All rights reserved. Used by permission.

24 Music by Gus Edwards, lyrics by Edward Madden, published in 1909.

25 These words are written in the old testament, which is called the Torah and is used in the Jewish religion.

26 Sigmund Freud, LL.D., *Witz und seine Beziehungen zum Unbewussten* [Wit and Its Relation to the Unconscious], New York, Moffat, Yard & Co., 1916.

27 Sam Fazio PhD, Director, Medical and Scientific Relations at the Alzheimer's Association Pennsylvania, 'Respectful adult communication improves quality of care in Alzheimer's', paper presented at the 2008 Alzheimer's Association International Conference on Alzheimer's Disease (ICAD 2008) Chicago.

28 Kristine Williams RN PhD, University of Kansas School of
     Nursing.
29 Access Economics, 'Dementia Estimates and Projections: Australian
     states and territories', Alzheimer's Australia, Canberra, 2005.
30 Joshua S. Rubinstein, David E. Meyers and Jeffrey E. Evans,
     'Executive control of cognitive processes in task switching', *Journal
     of Experimental Psychology: Human Perception and Performance*, vol. 27,
     no. 4, 2001, pp. 763–797.

RESOURCES

Important phone numbers

National Dementia Helpline: 1800 100 500
Interpreter services: 131 450
Alzheimer's Australia, national office: (02) 6254 4223
Carers Australia, national office: (02) 6282 7886

Dementia Care Australia

PO Box 378
Moorbank, Vic, 3138
Ph: (03) 9727 2744
Fax: (03) 3727 2766
www.dementiacareaustralia.com
At the 8th International IAHSA Conference in London in July 2009, Jane Verity, founder and president of Dementia Care Australia (DCA), and Hilary Lee, vice president of The Spark of Life, accepted the 2009 IAHSA Excellence in Ageing Services Award for The Spark of Life Culture Enrichment Program.

Alzheimer's Australia

PO Box 4019
Hawker, ACT, 2614
Ph: (02) 6254 4233
www.alzheimers.org.au

NSW Alzheimer's Association

Level 1, 40–50 Talavera Road,
Macquarie Park, NSW, 2113
PO Box 6042,
North Ryde, NSW, 2113
Ph: (02) 9805 0100
Fax: (02) 8875 4665
www.alzheimers.org.au

Alzheimer's New Zealand, national office

Level 3, Adelphi Finance House,
15 Courtenay Place,
PO Box 3643
Wellington, 6140
Ph: (04) 381 2362
Fax: (04) 381 2365
Email: nationaloffice@alzheimers.org.nz
www.alzheimers.org.nz

Alzheimer's Association, US

225 North Michigan Avenue,
Fl. 17, Chicago, Illinois 60601-7633
24-hour helpline: +1 1800 272 3900

Ph: +1 312 335 8700
Fax: +1 312 335 5886
Email: info@alz.org
www.alz.org

Alzheimer's Disease International

64 Great Suffolk Street,
London, SE1 0BL, United Kingdom
Ph: +44 20 7981 0880
Fax: +44 20 7928 2357
Email: info@alz.org.au
www.alz.co.uk

ACKNOWLEDGEMENTS

Bernard of Chartres, the twelfth-century philosopher, used to say that we are like dwarfs on the shoulders of giants, so that we can see more than they, and things at a greater distance, not by virtue of any sharpness of sight on our part, or any physical distinction, but because we are carried high and raised up by their giant size.

It is on the shoulders of the following people that I owe a tremendous gratitude for their part in the writing of this book.

To the generous and courageous spouses, children and loved ones of a person with dementia, thank you for agreeing to be interviewed and for sharing your personal experiences. Although your names have been changed to ensure your privacy I will never forget who you are.

To the staff at the Residential Care Unit whose patience, care and love blur the lines between human and angel, words cannot thank you enough. Thank you to the residents of the Residential Care Unit; each one of you has become a cherished member of my extended family.

To the gift of synchronicity bringing the beautiful Estelle Phillips into my life, who introduced me to the very special

Lynn Benjamin, who in turn introduced me to a true visionary, Maggie Hamilton. Thank you, Maggie, for believing in me before I had any idea I could write this book and for supporting me with your natural lightheartedness, love and joy.

To all those worked on the book my most heartfelt appreciation: Tricia Dearborn, Fiona Wilson, Clara Finlay, Emma Ward, Christa Moffitt, and my most patient, gracious and obliging editor, Aziza Kuypers, bless you. I could hear your gentle smile in every conversation.

To my darling friend, Judy Robinson, who always knows the right thing to say and to Debbie Uetz, whose story and courage helped me to say what needed to be said.

To Sheli Snir, who read and re-read every word of *Looking for Lionel*, offering me her invaluable critical support and editorial guidance. In your hand the pen is truly a sword. This book could not exist without you.

To Donna Jacobs Sife, who always knows how to make our mother laugh and sing and cry and feel completely adored. You are the most wonderful daughter, a truly inspirational sister, a devoted mother and a beautiful grandmother. Thank you for walking alongside me and supporting me to write our parents' story.

To Oren, soul mate, rock and father of our wonderful five children, every step we take together teaches me more about Love.

To my mother Lily who gave me the opportunity to choose Unconditional Love, and I did.

And finally to Lionel, thank you for being my dad. Thank you for the long conversations, the good times and bad, the Friday nights and Saturday breakfasts. Thank you for opening your heart at a time when keeping it shut might have hurt less but in doing so you healed all our hearts.